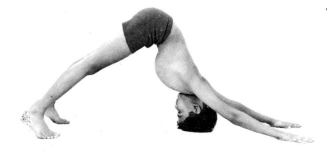

YOGA FOR CHILDREN

A Complete Illustrated Guide to Yoga

Including a Manual for Parents and Teachers

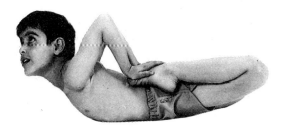

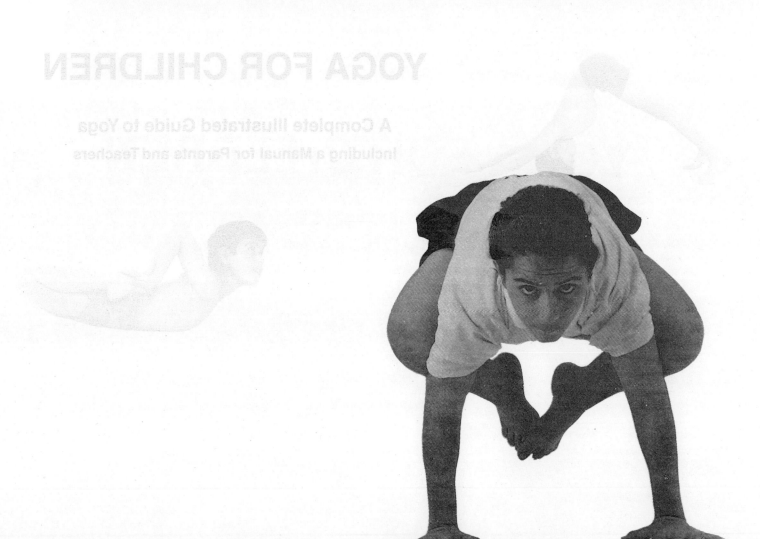

YOGA FOR CHILDREN

A Complete Illustrated Guide to Yoga

Including a Manual for Parents and Teachers

Swati Chanchani
Rajiv Chanchani

Design and Illustrations by J. Nath

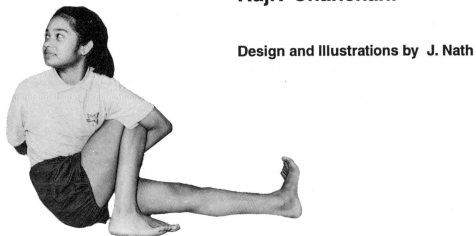

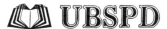 **UBSPD**

UBS Publishers' Distributors Ltd.

New Delhi ● Bangalore ● Chennai ● Calcutta ● Patna ●
Kanpur ● London

UBS Publishers' Distributors Pvt. Ltd.

5 Ansari Road, New Delhi-110 002
Phones: 3273601, 3266646 • Cable: ALLBOOKS • Fax: 3276593, 3274261
E-mail: ubspd@gobookshopping.com • Website: www.gobookshopping.com

10 First Main Road, Gandhi Nagar, Bangalore-560 009
Phones: 2253903, 2263901, 2263902 • Cable: ALLBOOKS
Fax: 2263904 • E-mail: ubspd.bng@bgl.vsnl.net.in

No. 60, Nelson Manickam Road, Chennai-600 029
Cable: UBSIPUB • E-mail: ubspd.che@md4.vsnl.net.in

8/1-B, Chowringhee Lane, Kolkata-700 016
Phones: 2441821, 2442910, 2449473 • Cable: UBSIPUBS
Fax: 2450027 • E-mail: ubspdcal@calvsnl.net.in

5 A, Rajendra Nagar, Patna-800 016
Phones: 672856, 673973, 686170 • Cable: UBSPUB • Fax: 686169
E-mail: ubspdpat1@sancharnet.in

80, Noronha Road, Cantonment, Kanpur-208 004
Phones: 369124, 362665, 357488 • Fax: 315122
E-mail: ubsknp@sancharnet.in

Distributors for Western India:
M/s Preface Books
Unit No. 223 (2nd floor), Cama Industrial Estate,
Sun Mill Compound, Lower Parel (W), Mumbai-400 013
Phone: 022-4988054 • Telefax: 022-4988048 • E-mail: Preface@vsnl.com

Overseas Contact:
475 North Circular Road, Neasden, London NW2 7QG, UK
Tele: (020) 8450-8667 • Fax: (020) 8452 6612 Attn: UBS

© Swati Chanchani & Rajiv Chanchani

First Published	1995
First Reprint	1995
Fourth Reprint	1998
Fifth Reprint	1999
Sixth Reprint	2000
Seventh Reprint	2000
Eighth Reprint	2001
Ninth Reprint	2002

Cover Design: UBS Art Studio.

Printed at Book Kraft, Delhi

Dedicated to
our revered teachers
Yogacharya B.K.S. Iyengar
Smt. Geeta Iyengar
Sri Prashant Iycngar

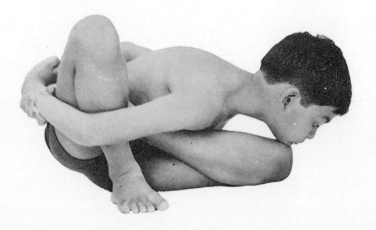

Acknowledgements

The authors thank Srineet Sridharan, Zarina Kolah, Anjali Nandi, Nachiket Chanchani and students at the Welham Girls High School for posing for the photographs, and Shri Subhash Patil and Shri Homyar Mistry for taking the photographs. We thank Lauren Fogel for proof reading the manuscript.

The manual for parents and teachers has been inspired by an unpublished article titled "Yoga For School Children" by Smt. Geeta Iyengar. With the author's permission we have reproduced parts of this article where appropriate.

Finally, we are ever grateful to the sisters of C.P.S..Ashram for constantly supporting us on the path of Yoga.

Foreword

I was, indeed, delighted to go through the typescript of *Yoga for Children*, written by Rajiv and Swati Chanchani. Both of them have been my pupils for a long time and have practised yoga regularly and sincerely.

After having observed at our Pune institute the techniques of imparting the knowledge of Yoga asanas to children, the authors began teaching Yoga to children first under the auspices of the Bharatiya Vidya Bhavan at Kodaikanal, Tamil Nadu, and later on their own.

On the basis of experience in teaching Yoga to children between the ages of 7 and 18, and keeping in view the specific problems or difficulties faced by them, the authors have undertaken the task of putting their perceptions in a book form.

As I read the text, I observed the interesting and exhilarating way in which the authors have explained the eight-limbs of yoga. They have also introduced seventy five asanas along with relevant stories to educate and motivate children to build up an ideal character and to improve their physical health and mental well-being.

Nature has gifted children with the ability to quickly recover from injuries. Hence, teachers need not be afraid while teaching them asanas. Moreover, they have an in-built instinct which helps them to react instantly to avoid injuries and muscular damage. They love speed and variety. If children are made to perform these asanas with different combinations and permutations, they get inspired to do more and more.

In addition to the qualities of speed and variety, children are also blessed with innocence and freshness. There is no jealousy or malice in them. Through Yoga, it is possible to transform skillfully their vanity and competitive spirit into useful forms of energy. Yoga channelises their thoughts and makes them responsible citizens of the world.

I am glad that two of my pupils have taken the initiative and brought out this book with stories and diagrams to convey the message of each asana on an educative level. These asanas can easily be taught in schools on a mass scale as well as in small groups at home or in clubs.

For children, who are custodians of each nation in particular and the whole world at large, I feel Yoga is the essential product of the twenty first century to lead them to perfect physical health and mental well-being.

B.K.S IYENGAR

Contents

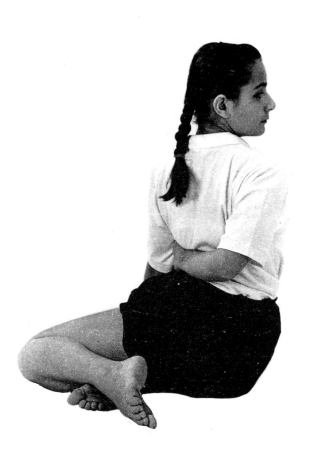

A Manual for
Parents and Teachers

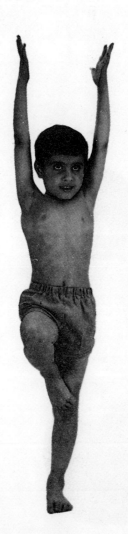

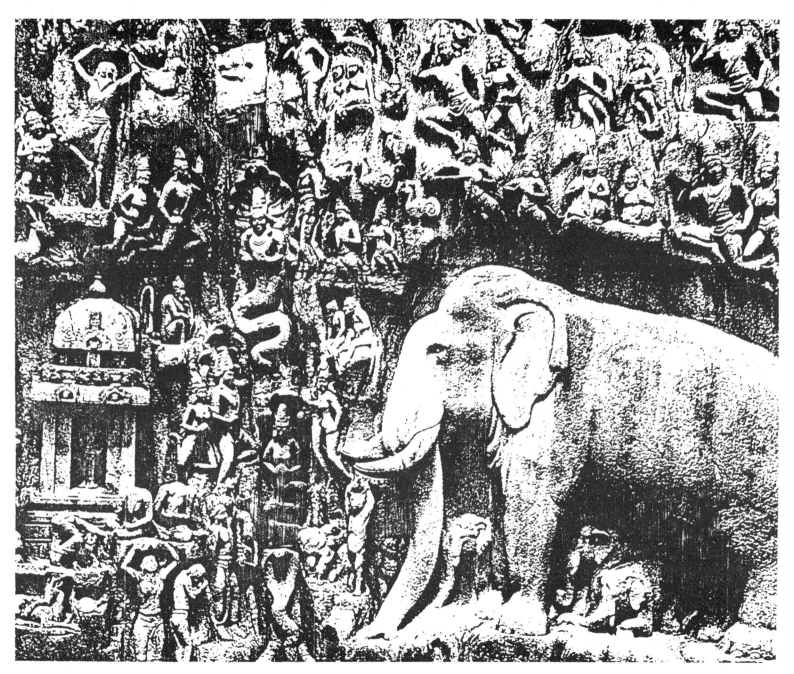

The penance of Sage Bhagirath, Mahabalipuram, Tamil Nadu

The Beginning

Yoga is an ancient science. Nobody knows its origins. Legends say it began with the gods. Lord Shiva is described as the first great yogi. Overtime many wise men walked the great path of Yoga. Each one of them left their own landmarks for us to follow.

Many old Indian stories tell us about these virtuous sages and their wonderful world. These sages were like children. Everything fascinated them: shining stars, tall mountains, flowing rivers, fierce beasts, beautiful birds....even little grasshoppers.

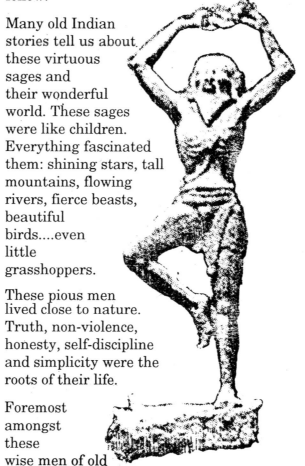

These pious men lived close to nature. Truth, non-violence, honesty, self-discipline and simplicity were the roots of their life.

Foremost amongst these wise men of old was the great Sage Patanjali.

Sage Patanjali

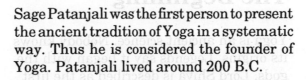

Sage Patanjali was the first person to present the ancient tradition of Yoga in a systematic way. Thus he is considered the founder of Yoga. Patanjali lived around 200 B.C.

There is an interesting story about Patanjali's birth. His mother, Gonika, was a very pious lady. One day while bathing in the river, Gonika prayed to the sun god, "O Lord, please grant me a glorious son."

In answer to her prayers the sun god told the wise snake Shesha (or Ananta) to take birth as Gonika's son. Instantly the great

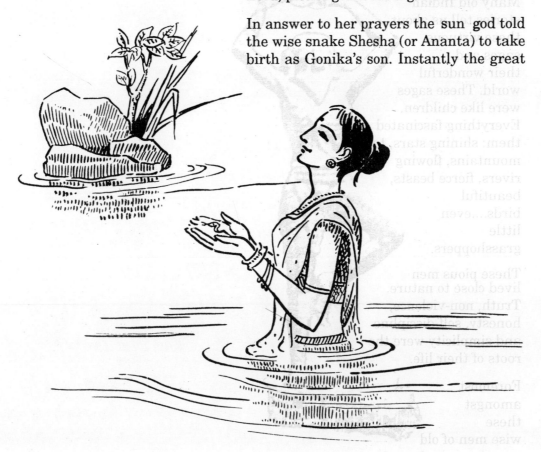

Shesha became a tiny snake and dropped down into Gonika's palms which were folded in prayer. The snake then changed himself into a beautiful baby boy. Gonika was delighted. She named the child Pata-anjali. Pata means falling and anjali means palms folded in prayer.

Patanjali grew up to be an extraordinary man, renowned for his learning and wisdom. He was the author of three brilliant works. One was on Sanskrit grammar. The second was a work on ancient Indian medicine, Ayurveda.

The third and the most important, was on Yoga. It is called the *Yoga Sutras of Patanjali*. In this brief work, containing only 196 sayings, Patanjali clearly explains what Yoga is.

Yoga Sutras of Patanjali

The Meaning of Yoga

The word Yoga means to join or unite. In the Yoga Sutras, Patanjali described Yoga as the means by which our mind can be made still, quiet and free from all distractions.

The Goal of Yoga

Patanjali explained that when the mind is kept very calm and quiet for a long time in dhyana, we become united with God and attain salvation. When a person attains salvation he reaches the goal of Yoga. This goal is called samadhi or kaivalya.

Requirements for Yoga

Patanjali taught that we must practice Yoga very diligently and watchfully. Try to keep an even mind, in success or failure, he said. He also taught us to live simply and avoid temptation.

The great sage further advised that we must cultivate good character traits. Be friendly, kind and compassionate, he taught. Be cheerful. Do not look for faults in others but always try to improve yourself.

Problems on the Path of Yoga

The wise Patanjali was careful to point out the obstacles that we may face while following the path of Yoga. He warned us to beware of ignorance, self importance, anger, hatred and excessive attachment. He explained that sickness, laziness, doubt and lack of concentration are all hurdles on this path.

The Path of Yoga

To enable us to cultivate the good qualities, and overcome the hurdles, Patanjali laid down an eight-fold path. This unique path is known as the Ashtanga-Yoga of Patanjali. A person who follows this path is called a yogi.

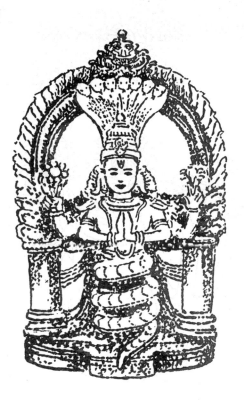

योगेन चित्तस्य पदेन वाचां
मलं शरीरस्य च वैद्यकेन।
योऽपाकरोत् तं प्रवरं मुनीनां
पतञ्जलिं प्राञ्जलिरानतोऽस्मि॥

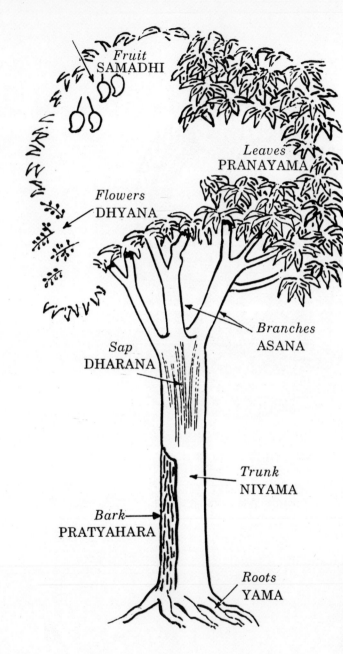

Fruit
SAMADHI

Leaves
PRANAYAMA

Flowers
DHYANA

Branches
ASANA

Sap
DHARANA

Trunk
NIYAMA

Bark
PRATYAHARA

Roots
YAMA

Ashtanga Yoga - The Eight-Fold Path

Ashta means eight and anga means limbs or parts. The eight limbs of Yoga are:

1. Yama   Yama refers to the Great Universal Commandments. Patanjali lists five yamas:

Ahimsa	- Non-violence
Satya	- Truth
Asteya	- Non-stealing
Brahmacharya	- Self-control
Aparigraha	- Unselfishness

2. Niyama   Niyama refers to personal disciplines. Patanjali lists five of these:

Saucha	- Cleanliness
Santosha	- Contentment
Tapas	- Great effort
Svadhyaya	- Self-study
Ishvara Pranidhana	- Faith in God

3. Asana   Asana means posture, such as the ones described in this book.

4. Pranayama   Pranayama means breath control.

5. Pratyahara   Pratyahara means control of the senses (taste, touch, smell, sight and hearing).

6. Dharana   Dharana means concentration.

7. Dhyana   Dhyana means meditation.

8. Samadhi   Samadhi or kaivalya, is the goal of Yoga where in the yogi unites with God.

By following this eight-fold path a man gets health of body and control over his mind. He becomes wise and compassionate.

For children, however, only the first three steps of Yoga are important: yama, niyama and asana. These steps prepare a child for the higher steps of Yoga which they can practice when they are older.

Yama-*Ahimsa*

Ahimsa is the first of the yamas. Ahimsa means non-violence. Saintly men have always preached and practiced non-violence in thought, word and deed. Lord Buddha was one of the greatest teachers of non-violence. He could influence men and even wild beasts to become harmless and peaceful.

Once Lord Buddha was walking down the road followed by several disciples. Seeing him, his jealous cousin Devadatta, unleashed a drunken elephant hoping that it would trample the Buddha to death

As the rampaging elephant charged down the street people ran helter-skelter. The Buddha's disciples also begged their master to flee. The Buddha, however, remained calm and refused to run away. The enraged elephant was further annoyed at seeing the Buddha unperturbed and came charging straight at him.

The Buddha calmly raised his hand in a gesture of non-violence. The angry beast stopped dead in its tracks! It then humbly kneeled down before the Buddha.

Such was the power of Lord Buddha's non-violence.

Yama-*Satya*

Satya is the second yama. Satya means truthful, honest or virtuous. The life of King Harish-Chandra provides a very good example of a man devoted to satya.

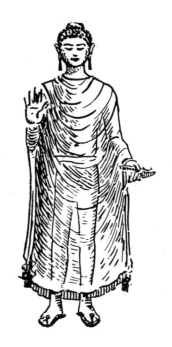

One day Sage Vasishtha met his rival, Sage Vishvamitra. "My disciple, King Harish-Chandra, is the most truthful man on earth," claimed Vasishtha.

"I shall prove that he is not," retorted Vishvamitra. Vishvamitra then promptly went to King Harish-Chandra's palace. In the guise of a poor brahmin he approached the king.. "O most generous King," he begged, "grant me two boons."

"You shall have whatever you want," said the large hearted Harish-Chandra.

"First, I want your kingdom and all your wealth," demanded the cunning brahmin.

Harish-Chandra was a man of his word. He willingly parted with everything he had and left for the forest clad in a single cloth. His wife and child followed him.

The brahmin was still not satisfied and followed them into the forest. "Harish-Chandra, now grant me my second wish."

"Pray, what more can I give you?" inquired the noble king.

"One and a half bushels of gold coins," demanded the greedy brahmin.

"Give me a month's time and I shall give you that too," promised Harish-Chandra.

The royal family then proceeded towards Kashi. Arriving there, Harish-Chandra

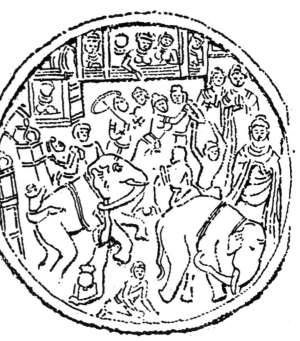

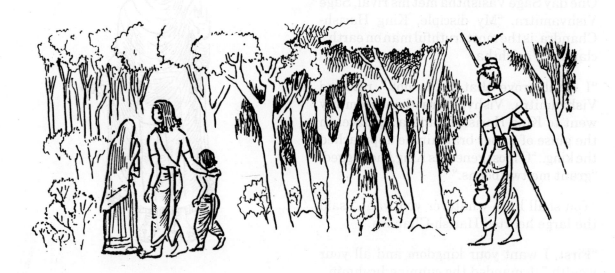

sought work but could find none. They were forced to beg for a living.

A month passed. The brahmin again appeared before Harish-Chandra, "Fulfill my second boon, O king, or accept that you are a liar," he said gleefully.

Seeing her husband's plight, the queen insisted, "Sell me as a slave, my lord, and fulfil your promise." Most reluctantly, Harish-Chandra agreed. He sold his wife and his son too, but still couldn't raise the required gold coins. He then sold himself and was finally able to fulfil his promise to the brahmin.

The queen and the prince had to toil long hours for a merchant. Still the merchant remained unsatisfied. Meanwhile, Harish-Chandra's master appointed him as an assistant in the crematorium.

Then one fateful day Harish-Chandra's son was bitten by a snake and died. The heartbroken mother carried the dead child to the crematorium. Harish-Chandra was shattered to see his wife bearing the dead body of their child. Still, he had to do his duty! "I am sorry, my dear," he said tearfully, "I cannot cremate our son unless you pay the cremation fees required by my master.

"My lord, I am a penniless slave," cried his wife.

In despair the couple decided to kill themselves. Harish-Chandra made a pyre of half-burnt logs. They placed their dead child on it. Then, seating themselves besides their child, they set the pyre ablaze.

At that moment Brahma, Indra and several other gods descended from heaven and doused the fire. "Harish Chandra," exclaimed the gods, "You have proved beyond doubt that you are the most honest man on earth. Your trials are over."

The gods brought the prince back to life and blessed the royal couple. Then Vishvamitra returned the kingdom to the virtuous and truthful King Harish-Chandra.

Yama-*Asteya*

Asteya is the third yama. Asteya means non-stealing. Sage Patanjali taught that to rob or steal is wrong. Even to be envious of what another owns is incorrect. The epic Ramayana provides a good example of a man who devotedly practiced the principle of asteya. His name was Prince Bharata.

Bharata's father, King Dasaratha, was the ruler of Ayodhya. Dasaratha had three wives. The eldest wife, Kausalya, was the mother of the crown prince Rama. The youngest wife, Sumitra, had two sons, Lakshmana and Shatrughana. The middle wife, Kaikeyi, was the mother of Prince Bharata.

Once while Prince Bharata was away at his grandfather's house, his mother, Queen Kaikeyi, learned that Prince Rama was to be crowned the king soon. This upset her. She went to her husband King Dasaratha, and said, "Grant me the two boons you had promised me years ago."

"Certainly, my beloved," replied the king

"First," said the ambitious Kaikeyi, "let my son Bharata be crowned king. And, banish Rama to the forest for fourteen years."

King Dasaratha was heart-broken at Kaikeyi's cruel demands. However, he was bound by his promise and granted Kaikeyi her boons.

The obedient prince Rama left for the forest accompanied by his wife, Sita, and brother, Lakshmana. Urgent summons were sent to Prince Bharata to return. Meanwhile, the aged King Dasaratha died of grief.

As Bharata entered Ayodhya he noticed the down-cast faces of the people. "Something is seriously wrong," he thought to himself as he rushed to his mother's chamber. Kaikeyi was delighted to see her son. "O Bharata," she proclaimed, you shall be crowned the king of Ayodhya! Your father is no more, and I have had Rama banished to the forest for fourteen years."

The good Bharata was horrified at his mother's words. "Mother", he cried, "You are blinded by greed.! I have no use for power, nor do I wish to rob my brother, Rama, of his kingdom!" Bharata immediately left for the forest. "I must bring my beloved brother Rama back to rule his kingdom," he resolved.

In the Chitrakuta forest Bharata met up with Rama, Sita and Lakshmana. Falling at Rama's feet, the pure hearted Bharata sobbed, "Forgive me, dear brother. I am innocent. Please return to govern your land and people. Our father, the king, is no more."

Rama knew that Bharata was faultless, but he could not be persuaded to come out of exile.

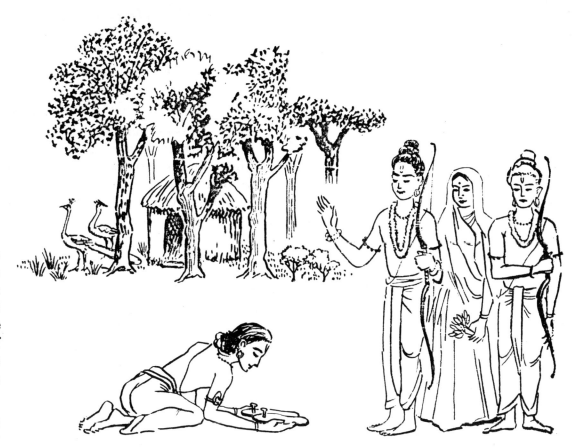

Finally, the wise sage Vashishtha intervened. He ordained that Bharata should serve as the king during Rama's absence.

With a heavy heart Bharata agreed. Before departing Bharata begged Rama to give him his sandals. On returning to Ayodhya, Bharata humbly placed Rama's sandals on the throne. He then moved to a hermitage on the outskirts of Ayodhya. Living the simple life of an ascetic, he ruled the kingdom from there.

When Rama returned from exile after fourteen years, the pure-hearted Bharata gladly handed over the kingdom to Lord Rama.

Yama-Brahmacharya

Brahmacharya is the fourth yama. Brahmacharya means self-control or self-discipline. A disciplined student who studies the scriptures is called a brahmachari.

Sage Vyasa's son, Shuka, was a great brahmachari. As a young boy, Shuka's father sent him to study under sage Brihaspati. Shuka was a keen and intelligent student and mastered many subjects. When Shuka returned home he continued to study and pray.

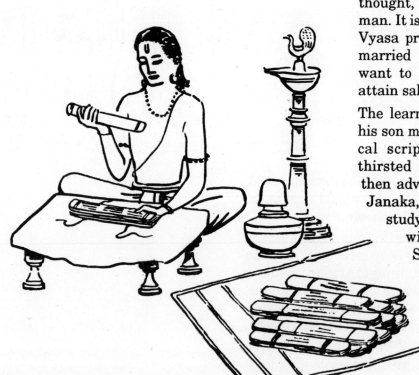

A few years passed, Sage Vyasa thought, "Shuka is now a young man. It is time for him to marry." Vyasa proposed that Shuka get married but he replied, "No, I want to become a sanyasi and attain salvation."

The learned sage Vyasa taught his son many further philosophical scriptures. Still, Shuka thirsted for knowledge. Vyasa then advised his son, "Seek out Janaka, the king of Mithila, and study under him. He is the wisest man on earth." Shuka set off for the distant kingdom. He journeyed over mountains and through forests for two years. Finally, Shuka arrived at Janaka's palace.

Through his yogic powers, King Janaka already knew of Shuka's arrival and the purpose of his visit. He decided to test Shuka. He instructed the sentries not to honour or welcome Shuka at the palace gates. Shuka was made to wait for three days. He waited patiently, undisturbed by this unkind reception.

On the fourth day Janaka arrived at the gates, welcomed Shuka and led him to the guest room. There Shuka was provided with every comfort. He was bathed in perfumed water, dressed in silken robes and given delicious food. Shuka showed no greed or great delight at these luxuries. Instead, he spent his days in meditation and prayer.

Because neither insults nor luxuries affected Shuka, King Janaka decided to put him to one final test. In the splendid court room, filled with dazzling performers, King Janaka gave Shuka a bowl full of milk. "Make seven rounds of this hall without spilling one drop of milk," said the King. Shuka accepted the bowl. He walked effortlessly around the great hall seven times, past the magnificient courtiers, the whirling dancing girls and the musicians, without spilling a single drop of milk.

King Janaka was delighted. "Shuka," he said, "You are unequalled in your self-control and self-discipline. I have nothing to teach you. Continue your practices and you will attain the supreme enlightenment."

Yama-*Aparigraha*

Aparigraha is the fifth yama. Aparigraha means not to grasp or clutch onto things. One should not be greedy and should learn to live with few possessions. Many years ago in South India there lived a pious brahmin named Vishnu-dasa. His life provides a good example of a man who firmly practised aparigraha.

Vishnu-dasa lived during the reign of the devout King Chola of Kanchi. King Chola prided himself on his piety. He offered fresh flowers and pearls to the gods in his daily worship.

One day while the king was offering his prayers, the simple Vishnu-dasa arrived at the temple. Unmindful of the king, he sat down to pray. During his worship, Vishnu-dasa offered the gods a few holy basil leaves and some clear, fresh water from an earthen pot.

Seeing this the proud king was offended, "You poor brahmin, how dare you offer the Lord such meagre offerings? You shall never attain the kingdom of heaven."

"Let us see who attains the kingdom of the gods first," replied Vishnu-dasa.

On returning to his palace, the king called his minister and asked, "What shall I do to please the gods?"

"Why not make a grand charitable home for the needy and the poor, your Honour?"

"That's an excellent idea. Let the work commence immediately commanded the king"

The pious Vishnu-dasa meanwhile continued to live an austere life devoted to prayer and worship. He lived simply and ate only one meal a day.

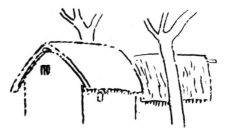

One day after completing his prayers, the poor brahmin, Vishnu-dasa, cooked his food and left it to cool on the window. He then went out for a short walk. When he returned he found that someone had eaten his food. The next day the same thing happened. The thefts continued daily. Deprived of his daily meal Vishnu-dasa thought, "Perhaps the gods want me to fast."

A few days later, while Vishnu-dasa was walking around as his food cooled, he noticed a ragged beggar creeping up to the window. As Vishnu dasa watched unobserved, he saw a hungry wretch stuffing food into his mouth and then sneaking away.

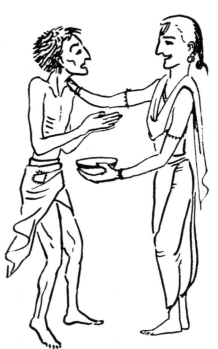

Vishnu-dasa felt very sorry for the starved beggar. Noticing that the beggar had left the butter uneaten, Vishnu-dasa ran after him, "Please wait," shouted Vishnu-dasa, "you have forgotten to eat the butter!" But the beggar ran faster, thinking that Vishnu-dasa wanted to beat him.

At last, Vishnu-dasa caught up with the beggar. "Do eat the butter, too," pleaded the selfless brahmin. The beggar was astonished to see the thin and frail brahmin parting happily with his food.

In an instant, the beggar changed into his true form. He was none other than the great Lord Vishnu! "My dear devotee, your selflessness is unmatched on earth," said Lord Vishnu. The Lord then took Vishnu-dasa to heaven.

Niyama-*Saucha*

Saucha is the first of the niyamas. Saucha means purity or cleanliness. Pure thoughts, good feelings and the cleanliness of the body are all aspects of saucha. While bathing and personal hygiene constitute external cleanliness, the practice of asanas and pranayama helps us cleanse our organs of toxins and impurities and our minds of impure thoughts. Yogis and devout people always purified themselves before commencing their prayers and daily activities.

A long time ago there lived a powerful king in Kashmir. Unfortunately, he contracted leprosy. Physicians and healers were called from far and wide to cure the king, but none of them succeeded.

The king then decided to go on a pilgrimage. He journeyed far and wide and met many holy men and sages, but none could help him. At long last he arrived at the temple town of Chidambaram. To purify himself before entering the shrine the king took a dip in the temple tank.

When he stepped out of the water, the king noticed that his body had been cleansed of the dreaded disease. His deformities were removed and his whole body sparkled with health and vigour.

The king's joy knew no bounds. Pure in body and mind he offered his thanks to Lord Shiva in the ancient temple. He then made a generous grant whereby the ancient temple was enlarged and made more glorious.

Niyama-*Santosha*

Santosha is the second niyama. Santosha means satisfaction or contentment. The story of Krishna and his childhood friend Sudama teaches us the meaning of santosha or contentment.

When Krishna was a young boy he studied at the ashram of Guru Sandipani. Krishna's best friend at the ashram was a clever brahmin boy named Sudama. The two boys studied, played and grew up together at the ashram.

On completing their studies the boys were sad to part. After leaving the ashram Krishna had many adventures. He eventually became the king of Dwaraka. Sudama chose to become a priest.

In time, Sudama married a devout lady named Sushila. Over the years Sudama's family grew but his earnings as a priest remained meagre. Sushila found it very difficult to make ends meet. One day there was no food in the house. In despair, Sushila turned to her husband.

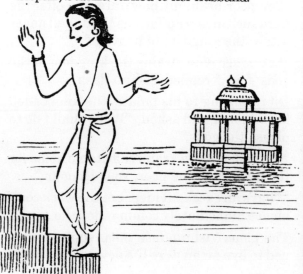

"Our children are hungry and crying. Why don't you go and see your childhood friend, Krishna. He is now the king of Dwaraka and will certainly help you."

Sudama's heart lit up at the thought of seeing his beloved friend. "I would love to see Krishna, he said, "but I shall not beg money from him."

Sushila was very happy. She borrowed some puffed rice from a neighbour and tied it into a cloth bundle. "Take this gift for your friend," she said.

Bearing the humble gift, Sudama set off for distant Dwaraka. After a long walk he arrived at Krishna's capital. The grandeur of the city overwhelmed him. Meekly, he walked up to the palace gates.

A sentry barred his way. "Who are you and what do you want?"

"I am Sudama." I have come to see my friend, King Krishna.

The guard couldn't believe that this poor man could be the king's friend. Reluctantly, he conveyed the message to the king.

Krishna was overjoyed to hear that Sudama had come to see him. He rushed to the palace gates to greet his dear friend. Embracing the weary Sudama, Krishna took him into the palace. The king himself washed Sudama's feet and saw to all his comforts.

Suddenly Krishna noticed the cloth bundle that Sudama had brought. "What is in that?" he asked.

Sudama felt ashamed to offer the king his modest present, but Krishna grabbed it from him and eagerly opened it. "Puffed rice," he said, "my favourite!" and began to eat handfuls of this simple fare.

Sudama was pleased to see that his friend, the king, was satisfied with his humble gift. The two friends talked for hours. At Krishna's request Sudama spent a few days at the palace. Finally, remembering that his family would be waiting for him, Sudama took his leave.

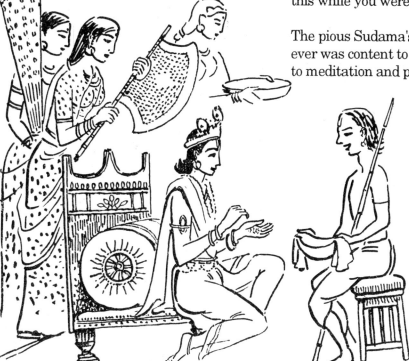

While returning in the royal chariot, Sudama remembered the purpose for which Sushila had sent him. "Krishna did not even ask me about my needs," he thought, "how can I return to my family empty handed?"

Downcast, Sudama got off the chariot a short distance from his hut. Sadly, he walked homewards. Strangely, a large mansion stood where his little hut had been. Sudama was worried. "Where is my little house?" he thought, "and where is my family?"

Just then Sushila opened the door. She was dressed in fine clothes and attended by many servants. "Welcome my Lord!" she greeted her husband joyously. "King Krishna arranged all this while you were away."

The pious Sudama's trials were over. He however was content to live a simple life dedicated to meditation and prayer.

Niyama-*Tapas*

Tapas is the third niyama. Tapas means penance, austerity or a burning effort.

The boy Dhruva is remembered for the difficult penance he practised.

Dhruva's father, the mighty king Uttanapada, had two wives. The elder wife, Suniti was kind and modest. Her son was Dhruva. The younger wife, Surichi was haughty and ambitious. She was the mother of Uttama.

Surichi was the king's favourite. She wished to ensure that her son would be the king's successor. She therefore, took every opportunity to belittle the elder queen and her innocent son Dhruva. The king believed Surichi's tales and showered all his affection on the younger queen and her son.

One day little Dhruva, finding his father alone, went and sat on his lap. At that moment Surichi arrived, "How dare you sit on the king's lap?" she screamed and pulled Dhruva out of his father's lap.

Dhruva was hurt and went crying to his mother. "Mother," he vowed, "I shall practice penance and attain a position higher than that of my father, the king!"

Suniti tried to dissuade her son, but the strong-willed boy held steadfastly to his vow. Finally, Dhruva obtained his mother's blessings and left for the forest

Although he was only a boy, Dhruva wandered alone in the forest in search of a teacher. Whenever Dhruva met wise and holy men he asked them, "Please, can you show me the path to heaven?"

Some wisemen admired his courage, others laughed at him, and others asked him to return home. None, however, could show him the path sought.

The unwavering Dhruva continued his search. He lived on wild fruits, berries and water. Neither heat nor cold, neither wild beasts nor hunger could deter him from his efforts. Then one day Dhruva met the wise sage, Narada. Narada taught Dhruva a prayer. "If you wish to reach heaven," said Narada, "chant this prayer and meditate on the Lord."

Dhruva was happy for the guidance. He sat cross-legged under a tree and concentrated his thoughts and feelings on Lord Vishnu. For days on end he mediated, prayed and fasted.

Greatly impressed by the child's burning efforts and austerities, Lord Vishnu appeared before him.

"O Lord," the boy prayed, "please remove all my mother's sorrows and grant me a place in heaven."

"Dhruva", said Lord Vishnu. "Your penance has been more severe than that of great sages. I shall grant your wish. Now, return home to your mother."

Young Dhruva returned home with a large following. His parents were delighted to see him. Surichi apologised for having mistreated him.

When Dhruva came of age, King Uttanapada crowned him king. Dhruva wisely governed his kingdom for many years. When he grew old Vishnu raised him to the heavens and made him a bright star called Dhruva, the pole star.

Niyama-*Svadhyaya*

Svadhyaya is the fourth niyama. Svadhyaya means self-study or to know one's self. In the Upanishads there is a story of young boy named Nachiketa. Nachiketa provides a good example of somebody who really wanted to know and understand himself.

Nachiketa's father, sage Vajashravasa, once conducted a great ceremony. In the hope that he would reach heaven he gave many cows for alms. However, these cows were lean and old. Nachiketa was saddened to see his father's lack of generosity.

To reprimand his father the little boy asked, "Who will you give me to, father?"

At first Vajashravasa did not reply. Nachiketa persisted with his question. Annoyed, his father muttered, "I give you to the God of Death."

Undaunted, Nachiketa marched off to the palace of Yama, the God of Death. Yama was away and so Nachiketa waited, fasting and praying in the meanwhile. Three days later, when Yama returned, he found a fearless boy standing at the palace gates. The God of Death was pleased with the lad's devotion and determination. "Since you have waited for three days I shall grant you three boons," he said to Nachiketa.

"Then let my father be happy when I return to him on earth." requested Nachiketa.

"Granted," answered Yama.

"Now tell me how to get to heaven?" asked Nachiketa.

Yama then taught Nachiketa how to attain the sorrowless world called heaven.

"And lastly," demanded Nachiketa, "explain to me what happens to a man after he dies."

"That is a very difficult question," said Yama, taken aback. "Ask for anything else, herds of cattle, many elephants, gold, palaces, a long life.

"Oh no, I don't want any of these things," insisted Nachiketa. "Tell me, does a man continue to exist after he dies?"

Convinced of Nachiketa's keen desire to understand the mysteries of life and death, Yama relented.

"The soul continues to exist though the body dies and decays," explained Yama.

"The soul is like a rider," continued Yama, "and your body is like a chariot. Your intelligence is the charioteer and your thoughts and feeling are the reins. Your five senses, sight, hearing, smell, taste and touch are the five horses that draw the chariot. The world around you is like the pastures on which these horses graze."

Then Yama taught Nachiketa the importance of yoga. He explained, "By practicing Yoga, Nachiketa, you can bring your senses under control just as a charioteer brings his horses under control. As soon as you have controlled your senses, you will see the soul and understand yourself."

Nachiketa learned well what Yama taught. He made a deep effort to understand his true nature and thereby became a wise and perfect man.

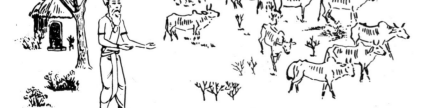

Niyama-Ishvara Pranidhana

Ishvara pranidhana is the last niyama. Ishvara pranidhana means faith in God. There is an amazing story of a boy named Prahlada who, though born of demon parents, had tremendous faith in God.

King Hiranya-kashyapu, who controlled a vast empire, was a powerful demon. He hated Lord Vishnu because Vishnu had killed his twin brother. One day he summoned his ministers and said, "Destroy all temples and images of Vishnu in my kingdom. Burn all books bearing Vishnu's name and make sure that no one chants his name in my domain!"

The king wished to ensure that his little boy, Prahlada, would grow up to be a fierce demon. Therefore, he entrusted Prahlada to a renowned teacher saying, "Initiate the boy into all the demonic ways, teach him to despise the gods and make sure he never hears the name of Vishnu."

Several months later, keen to know how his son had fared in his studies, the king sent for Prahlada, "Boy, what have you learned so far?"

"I have learned to adore the name of Vishnu," said the innocent child.

"What!" cried Hiranya-kashyapu, hardly able to believe his ears. "Call the boy's teacher and chop off his head!"

Trembling, the teacher arrived, "Pardon me, my Lord, I did not teach Prahlada to adore Vishnu."

"Then who taught you that dreadful name?" thundered Hiranya-kashyapu.

"Lord Vishnu himself taught me," replied the devout Prahlada.

"Take this boy away," fumed the king, "and rid him of this nonsense which he has learned."

Disillusioned, the king left Prahlada to his studies for a few more years. Then he once again summoned the boy.

"Now have you learned anything sensible?" he questioned his son.

"I bow to the great Lord Vishnu, began the pious boy.

Furious, the king ordered his demon soldiers to kill the boy. The soldiers attacked Prahlada with sharp-edged swords and heavy clubs. Prahlada stood calmly chanting the name of Lord Vishnu, and with the Lord's protection remained uninjured by the blows.

The enraged king then ordered his soldiers to throw Prahlada into a pit full of poisonous snakes. Prahlada stood fearlessly amidst the serpents, and chanting Lord Vishnu's name remained unharmed.

"Throw Prahlada into the fire, "commanded the infuriated king. But the devout Prahlada came out of the fire unscathed.

"Drown the boy in the ocean," ordered the wicked king. However, Lord Vishnu also protected Prahlada from drowning.

"Hurl Prahlada off a high cliff," said the cruel king. Even while Prahlada fell he continued mediating on Lord Vishnu. He landed gently on the ground and was unhurt. Prahlada then returned to his father's palace and continued his life of prayer and meditation.

One day as the faithful boy chanted his prayers, Hiranya-kashyapu challenged him "Since you say Vishnu is everywhere, show him to me in this pillar!"

With a terrible roar Lord Vishnu burst out of the pillar in the form of a half-man-half-lion. He killed the tyrannical king and blessed his little devotee.

The pious Prahlada was then crowned king.

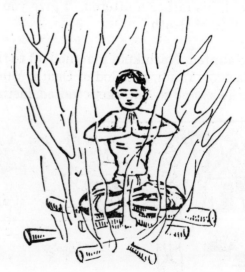

Asana

Asana is the third stage of Ashtanga-Yoga. Asana means a posture or a stance. Legends say that asanas originated from Lord Shiva.

Lord Shiva assumed different stances or asanas to create the different forms of life. Each time he performed an asana a new creature was born. As he did 84,000,000 asanas, 84,000,000 living species came into being. Yogis, however, know and practice only a few of these asanas.

While many asanas represent living things such as a tree, a fish or a crane, asanas have also been derived from other sources. A few asanas are derived from natural forms such as a mountain or the moon. Some asanas resemble man-made objects like a boat or a plough. Still others are dedicated to sages or the gods. Geometrical shapes have also inspired asanas, for example, the triangle-pose. The names of some other asanas refer to parts of the body.

Sage Patanjali taught that you should be firm and steady while performing an asana. Correct practice, he said, should lead to a feeling of well-being.

Asanas are scientific exercises. They not only make us strong and supple, but they also help to remove impurities from our bodies. By practicing asanas, the circulation, respiration, digestion and elimination are all improved. Asanas also improve the memory, concentration and will-power. They teach us how to be calm. Asanas are thus invaluable for the health of body and mind.

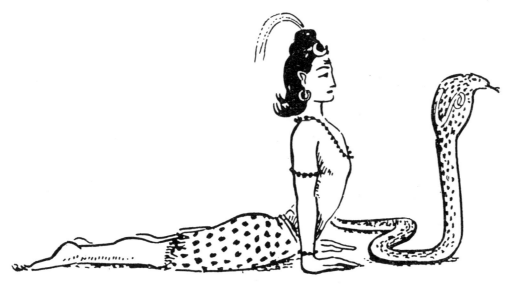

Pranayama

Pranayama is the fourth stage of Yoga. Pranayama means breath control. There are three important movements in pranayama inhalation of the breath, exhalation of the breath and retention of the breath.

There is an interesting story in the *Upanishads* which shows the importance of the breath.

Once there was a dispute between the eyes, the ears, the speech, the mind and the breath as to who was the most important. They all approached Lord Brahma and asked him, "Pray tell us, who is the greatest amongst us?"

"That's easy," Brahma said. "Each of you will leave the body for a year. The body will then decide who amongst you is the greatest."

Following Brahma's advice, first the tongue went off leaving the body without speech for a whole year. When the tongue came back the eyes went off leaving the body blind for a year. When the eyes returned, the ears went off leaving the body deaf for a year. When the ears returned, the mind went off and the body remained like a simpleton for a whole year. Then the mind returned.

Next it was the breath's turn to leave the body. As soon as the breath began to depart the tongue lost its power of speech, the eyes lost their power to see, the ears lost their ability to hear and the mind lost its intelligence! "Come back, come back, O breath," they prayed, "for you are the greatest amongst us!"

The breath then returned and the body became whole again.

Pratyahara

Pratyahara is the fifth stage of Ashtanga Yoga. Prayahara means to restrain or to withdraw. In pratyahara the yogi remains quiet. He does not get distracted or disturbed by things which he sees, hears, smells tastes or feels.

The great sage Chayavana provides a perfect example of someone who practised pratyahara. In his youth Chayavana retired to a peaceful place in the forest.

He sat down, closed his eyes and fixed his mind on God. Many days, weeks and seasons passed, but Chayavana did not feel or notice anything. He remained still and quiet. Years went by, white ants made a big mound over him. Plants and creepers covered the ant hill. Birds and little creatures made their homes amongst the vegetation and still Chayavana remained unmoving, unmindful of the changes around him.

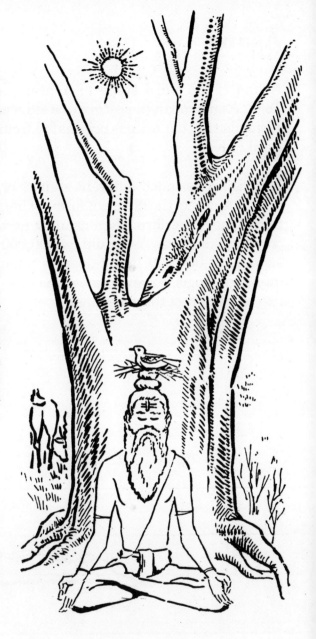

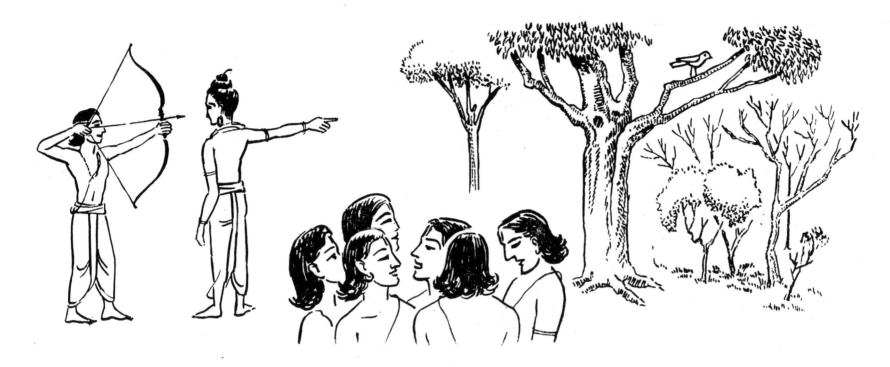

Dharana

Dharana is the sixth stage of Ashtanga Yoga. Dharana means keeping the mind steady and concentrated. Arjuna's reply to his guru Drona's question provides a fine example of dharana.

Once Guru Drona was instructing his pupils, the young Kaurava and Pandava princes, in the science of archery. For a target Drona placed a wooden bird on the branch of a distant tree. He then asked his pupils to come forward one by one to test their skill and concentration. First he called Yudhisthira.

"What do you see?" Drona **asked, pointing to** the target.

"Sir," replied Yudhisthira, "I see the blue sky, a tree, branches, leaves and a bird sitting amongst them."

"Go back and sit down," snapped Drona annoyed at this answer. "There is no way that you will be able to hit the target."

Then Drona called the other princes one by one, "What do you see there?" he asked each of them. The replies were similar to Yudhisthira's. "You are all unfit even to attempt to shoot this target," he said.

Finally, it was Arjuna's turn. "Well, what do you see there, Arjuna?" Drona addressed his favourite student.

Arjuna looked intently at the target. "Sir,' he said, "I see only the right eye of a bird."

Drona was pleased. "Good," he said, "now you must try and shoot the bird's eye."

Arjuna concentrated his mind on the target, took careful aim and lo! he pierced the bird's eye with his first arrow.

Delighted, Drona hugged his keen and attentive pupil.

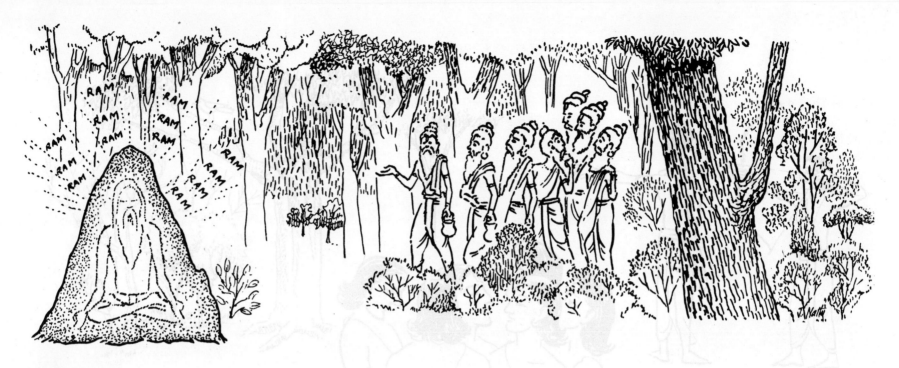

Dhyana

Dhyana is the seventh stage of Ashtanga Yoga. Dhyana means meditation, contemplation or reflection on God. The hermit Valmiki provides a good example of someone deeply absorbed in meditation.

Strangely, Valmiki was a bandit in his early life. One day he came upon the seven wise sages journeying through the forest. Valmiki demanded that they hand him any valuable they had.

The wise sages suggested that, Valmiki meet his family and ask them whether they would share his sins as they shared his plundered wealth. Valmiki ran to his family and put this question to them He was horrified when his wife and children refused to share the responsibility for his misdeeds.

Valmiki rushed back to the wise sages and sought their forgiveness. "Show me the path whereby I can become a good man," he begged.

The sages then asked him to chant "Mara," the name of the God of Death.

Immediately the robber sat down under tree and began to chant "Ma-ra, Ma-ra, Ma-ra." He chanted for a long time and gradually, as the rogue became purer his chant changed from "Ma-ra, Ma-ra, Ma-ra to Ra-ma, Ra-ma, Ra-ma." For years Valmiki continuously chanted Lord Rama's name.

White ants covered the meditating hermit under a mound of earth, still Valmiki remained absorbed in his meditation.

Many years later the seven sages again passed through the same forest. Thy heard the chant "Ra-ma, Ra-ma, Ra-ma," coming from an ant hill. When the sages broke the and hill they discovered Valmiki immersed in meditation. As they found him in a mound of white ants, valmika, they named him Valmiki.

Years later the wise sage Valmiki composed the great Ramayana.

Samadhi

Samadhi is the eighth and final stage of Ashtanga Yoga. In samadhi the mind is concentrated perfectly on God for a long time. The yogi then has a vision of God and becomes a wise and holy sage. Sage Kapila was a master of Yoga and showed several keen disciples the way to God.

When Kapila's father died, his mother, Devahuti, sought her son's guidance on the path of Yoga. Kapila knew that his mother was a devout and pious lady ready to receive the highest knowledge. So he taught her the advanced aspects of Yoga.

Devahuti then retired to the forest clad in garments made of bark. There she prayed and fasted. One day, while she sat in deep meditation on the banks of the river Sarasvati, Devahuti attained the goal of Yoga, samadhi! She then became one with God.

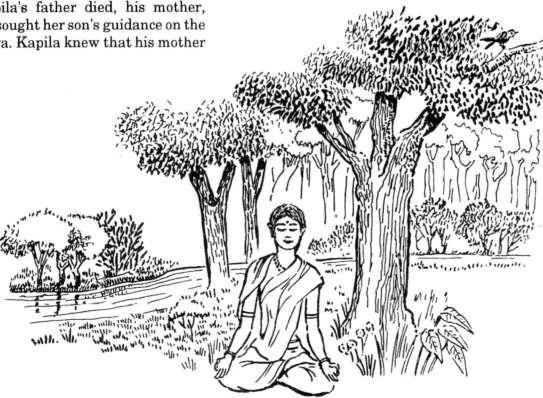

Important Dos and Don'ts

Place

Asanas should be practised in a clean, airy and well lit room. The floor should be level. If it is not possible to practise indoors, you may practise on level ground outdoors.

Time

The best time to practise asanas is in the morning before breakfast or in the evening before dinner.

Food

Do not practise asanas immediately after eating. Let two to four hours pass after eating a meal, and wait at least one or two hours after eating a snack.

Requirements

All you require for Yoga is a mat or a folded blanket.

Cleanliness

Take a bath if possible, and go to the toilet before you begin your practice. Do not wear shoes or socks while doing the asanas.

Sickness

When you are sick you must rest. If, however, you have a small problem such as a cold, a cough, a headache, a stomach ache, a sprained ankle, etc. then consult your teacher and seek his guidance. Remember that Yoga can help relieve your problems.

For Girls

When you have your menstrual period never do upside down poses such as Shirsha-asana. Sarvanga-asana, Hala-asana, Karna-pida-asana, Adho Mukha Vriksha-asana, etc.. You may do all the other poses. However, do consult your teacher.

Little Children

Children below 8 years will not be able to accurately perform asanas such as Shirsha-asana, Sarvanga-asana, Hala-asana and Karna-pida-asana and the asanas introduced in Course III, because their bodies have yet to develop. Do not force or tease the little children.

Timings

In this book each " count" is equal to approximately one second. You may perform each asana repeatedly two or three times before going on to the next one.

Breathing

Don't force yourself to breathe deeply or to hold your breath while doing the asanas. Breathe normally while doing the asanas. Always breathe through the nose.

Yoga mind

Always be alert attentive and watchful when you practice. Concentrate on your own pose. Watch your teachers carefully and pay attention to their instructions.

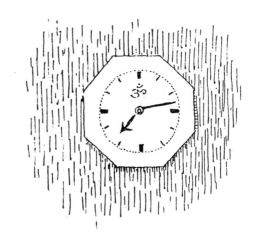

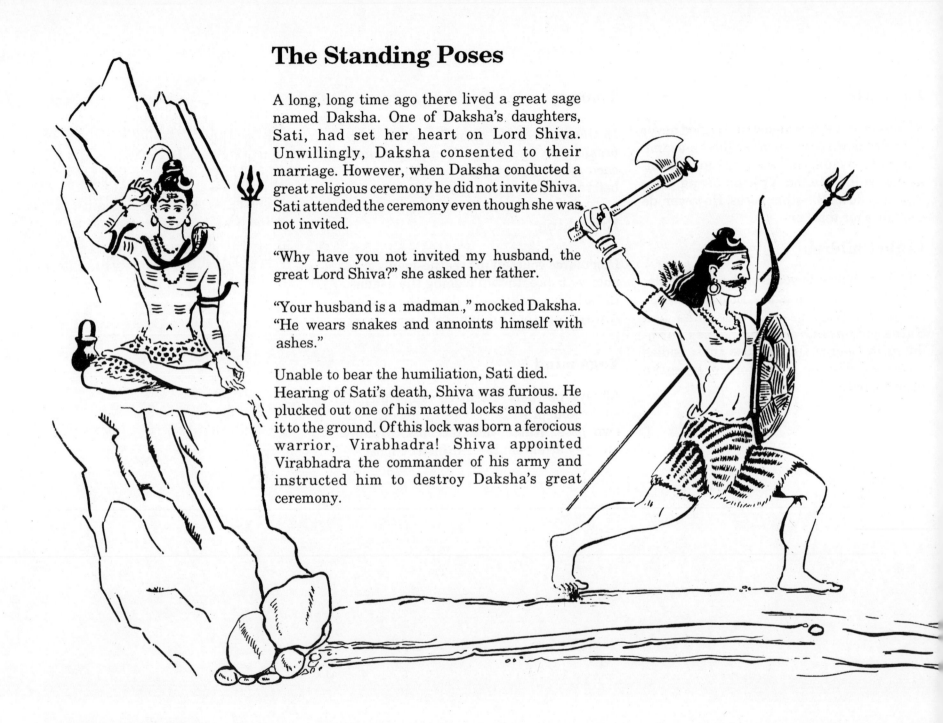

The Standing Poses

A long, long time ago there lived a great sage named Daksha. One of Daksha's daughters, Sati, had set her heart on Lord Shiva. Unwillingly, Daksha consented to their marriage. However, when Daksha conducted a great religious ceremony he did not invite Shiva. Sati attended the ceremony even though she was not invited.

"Why have you not invited my husband, the great Lord Shiva?" she asked her father.

"Your husband is a madman," mocked Daksha. "He wears snakes and annoints himself with ashes."

Unable to bear the humiliation, Sati died. Hearing of Sati's death, Shiva was furious. He plucked out one of his matted locks and dashed it to the ground. Of this lock was born a ferocious warrior, Virabhadra! Shiva appointed Virabhadra the commander of his army and instructed him to destroy Daksha's great ceremony.

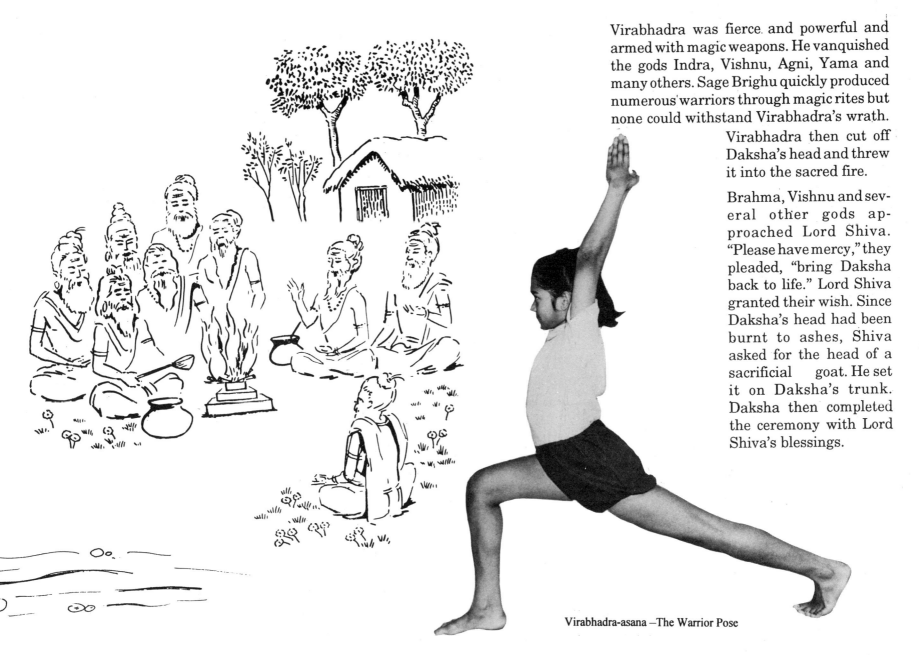

Virabhadra was fierce and powerful and armed with magic weapons. He vanquished the gods Indra, Vishnu, Agni, Yama and many others. Sage Brighu quickly produced numerous warriors through magic rites but none could withstand Virabhadra's wrath.

Virabhadra then cut off Daksha's head and threw it into the sacred fire.

Brahma, Vishnu and several other gods approached Lord Shiva. "Please have mercy," they pleaded, "bring Daksha back to life." Lord Shiva granted their wish. Since Daksha's head had been burnt to ashes, Shiva asked for the head of a sacrificial goat. He set it on Daksha's trunk. Daksha then completed the ceremony with Lord Shiva's blessings.

Virabhadra-asana —The Warrior Pose

1. Tada-asana
2. Urdhva Hasta-asana

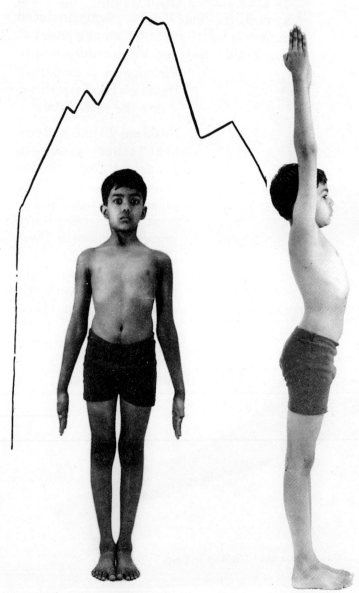

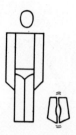
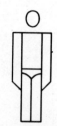
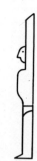

1. Stand straight. Join your feet. Keep your heels and bigtoes touching each other. Extend your arms downwards with your palms facing your thighs.

2. Tighten your knees and elbows. Broaden your chest. Draw your shoulders back. Look straight ahead. This is *Tada-asana*.

3. Stretch your arms overhead. Keep your palms facing each other. This is *Urdhva Hasta-asana*.

DO

○ Be firm and tall as a mountain.

○ Stand with equal weight on both your feet.

DON'T

☐ Don't protrude your buttocks.

☐ Don't hold your breath.

BENEFITS

✿ Teaches you to stand correctly.

✿ Makes the back straight and strong.

✿ Makes the mind alert.

Tada means mountain. The highest mountains are the Himalayas. Many Indians consider them sacred. The great god of Yoga, Lord Shiva, lives on a high Himalayan peak named Kailash. His wife Parvati, is the daughter of the Himalayas. Their son Ganesh is the remover of obstacles. Parvati's sister, the river Ganga, arises from the melting snows of a Himalayan glacier.

The Himalayas have always been a favourite retreat for Indian sages. They retired to these quiet and beautiful mountains to practise Yoga and do penance. Many great masters of Yoga attained wisdom in the Himalayas.

Urdhva means raised and hasta means arm. This is the raised-arm pose.

3. Vriksha-asana

10 to 15 counts each side

Vriksha means tree. Once upon a time all men were good and honest. In those days a magic wish-fulfilling tree called Kalpa Vriksha grew on earth. Men had no need for possessions as they could simply wish for whatever they desired. Over time men became wicked and dishonest, and so the magic tree was removed to Lord Indra's garden in heaven.

Don't ordinary trees also fulfill many of our wishes? They provide flowers, fruit, wood and shade. They serve as homes for birds and animals. Trees also protect the soil from erosion.

Like trees, Yoga-asanas also give many benefits. Health, strength, flexibility, concentration and grace are all fruits of a regular practice

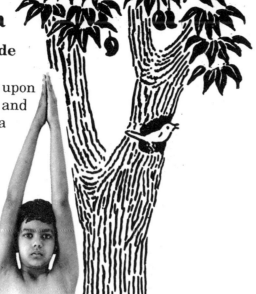

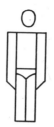

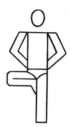

DO

○ Imagine you are a tall tree with deep roots.

1. Stand in Tada-asana.

2. Bend your right knee. Place your right foot on your left upper thigh. Rest your hands on your hips.

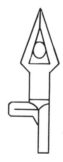

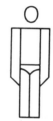

3. Stretch your arms up. Join your palms. This is *Vriksha-asana*.

DON'T

☐ Don't sway like a tree in the wind.

☐ Don't bring your bent-knee forward.

4. **Return** to Tada-asana. Now keep your **right leg straight** and bend your **left leg**. Do the pose on the other side.

5. **Then come back to Tada-asana.**

BENEFITS

✿ Strengthens the shoulders and legs.

✿ Improves concentration and balance.

4. Utkata-asana

5 to 15 counts

Utkata means high, mighty or superior. The great epic Ramayana tells that Rama's wife Sita was captured by Ravana, the king of Lanka. To rescue his wife, Rama made friends with the bears and monkeys. With a mighty leap, Hanuman, the great monkey, crossed the ocean and landed in Lanka. He found Sita but was captured by Ravana's soldiers.

Brought before Ravana, the monkey decided to teach the proud and wicked monarch a lesson. Using his magic power, he made his tail grow very long. He then coiled it into a high seat and sat upon it, looking down at the king. Angrily Ravana ordered, "Move my throne to a higher place." Instantly, Hanuman's magic tail grew and his seat rose higher than the king's throne. Furious, Ravana ordered, "Raise my throne to an even higher place." But Hanuman's magic seat rose higher still.

Enraged, Ravana ordered that Hanuman's tail be set on fire. Instead, Hanuman set Lanka on fire and escaped. So Hanuman showed that he was superior to the wicked King of Lanka.

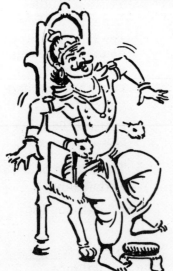

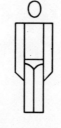

1. Stand in Tada-asana.

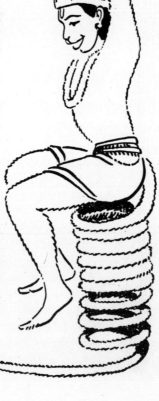

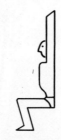

2. Stretch your arms upwards. Join your palms. Bend your knees. Look straight ahead. This is *Utkata-asana*. Then return to Tada-asana.

DO
○ Imagine you are sitting on a chair.

DON'T
☐ Don't lean forward.

BENEFITS
✿ Strengthens the ankles, calves, inner thighs and back.

5. Garuda-asana

10 to 15 counts each side

Garuda was born with the body of a man and the head, wings and claws of an eagle. He was the son of Vinata, the mother of all eagles. His mother had lost a bet to her sister, Kadru, the mother of all snakes. Vinata had thus become Kadru's slave.

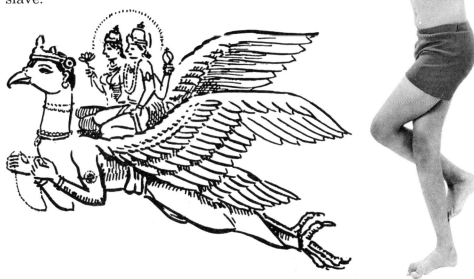

Garuda vowed to purchase his mother's freedom. The serpents demanded as ransom the nectar of immortality which lay with the gods. With his mother's blessings, Garuda flew to the heavens. There, in a fierce battle, he defeated Lord Indra, the Sun, the Moon and the lesser gods. He then lifted the pot of nectar in his beak and flew back.

On the return journey, Garuda met Lord Vishnu. Greatly impressed by Garuda's valour, Vishnu granted him a boon. Garuda asked that he be allowed to serve as Lord Vishnu's vehicle. He also asked for immortality. Vishnu granted these wishes.

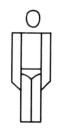

.. Stand in Tada-asana.

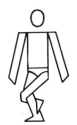

2. Bend your knees. Place your left leg over the right leg, and entwine it around.

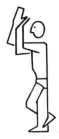

3. Bend your arms. Place one arm over the other, and entwine them around each other. This is *Garuda-asana*.

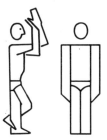

4. Return to Tada-asana. Now place your right leg over the left. Interchange the position of the arms. Repeat the pose. Finally return to Tada-asana.

DO
- Look straight ahead.

DON'T
- Don't entwine loosely.

BENEFITS
- Strengthens the ankles.
- Relieves cramps in the calves.

6. Utthita Trikona-asana

10 to 20 counts each side

Utthita means extended. Tri means three and kona means angle. Trikona means triangle. In fact, in this pose you make several triangles. Remember, triangles are formed by straight lines. So keep your limbs straight while doing Utthita Trikona-asana.

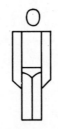

1. Stand in Tada-asana.

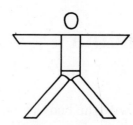

2. Jump and spread your legs 2 to 3 feet apart and your arms sideways. Stand on a line, toes pointing forward and palms turned down.

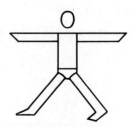

3. Turn your right foot out 90° and your left foot in slightly.

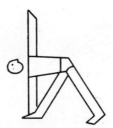

4. Bend sideways to your right. Place your right palm on your right ankle or the floor. Stretch your left arm up. Look up at your fingertips. This is *Utthita Trikona-asana*.

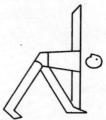

5. Come up. Return to position 2. Now turn your left foot out 90° and your right foot in slightly. Do the pose on the left side.

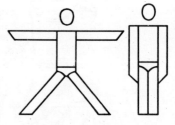

6. Come up. Return to position 2. Then jump back to Tada-asana.

DO

○ Align your head and hips on the line on which you are standing.

DON'T

☐ Don't bend your knees or your elbows.

BENEFITS

✿ Shapes the legs, strengthens the ankles.

✿ Improves the arches of the feet.

✿ Builds up the chest.

7. Parivritta Trikona-asana

10 to 20 counts each side

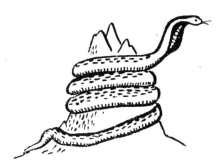

Parivritta means twisted or revolved and trikona means triangle. This is the twisted triangle pose. One day the snake king, Vasuki, had an argument with the wind god, Vayu. The snake wound himself around the three-peaked mountain Trikuta, so tightly that the wind couldn't even enter. Angrily, Vayu blew a cyclone which shook the earth and the heavens. Alarmed, Lord Vishnu told them to stop quarrelling. As Vasuki loosened his grip, the wind whisked away the mountain and dropped it into the southern sea.

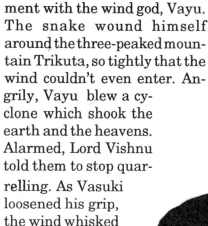

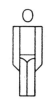

1. Stand in Tada-asana.

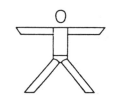

2. Jump and spread your legs 2 to 3 feet apart and your arms sideways. Stand on a line, toes pointing forward and palms turned down.

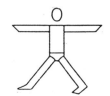

3. Turn your right foot out 90° and your left foot in 45°. Keep both legs poker stiff.

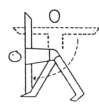

4. Rotate your waist and bring your left palm on your right ankle or the floor. Stretch your right arm up. Look up at your fingertips. This is *Parivritta Trikona-asana.*

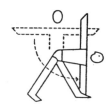

5. Come up. **Return to** position 2. Now **turn** your left foot **out and** your right in. **Do the** pose on the **left side.**

BENEFITS

✿ Helps straighten hunched **back and** rounded **shoulders.**

✿ Makes the **entire body** strong and elastic.

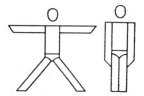

6. Come up. Return to position 2. Then jump back to Tada-asana.

DO

○ Narrow your waist, expand your chest.

○ Align your head and arms on a line.

○ Keep your head exactly above your ankle.

DON'T

☐ Don't let your thigh muscles loosen.

8. Utthita Parshva-kona-asana

10 to 20 counts each side

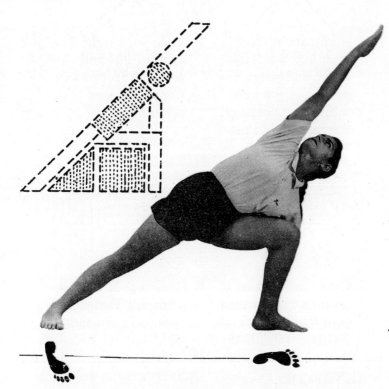

Utthita means stretched, parshva means side, and kona means an angle. By correctly stretching, bending and turning in Utthita Parshva-kona-asana you form several geometrical shapes: squares, triangles, and right angles.

Remember, right means achieve right ends. So spread your legs just the right distance to achieve the right angle of the bent-knee.

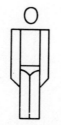

1. Stand in Tada-asana.

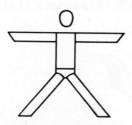

2. Jump and spread your legs 3 to 4 feet apart and your arms sideways. Stand on a line, toes pointing forward and palms facing down.

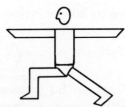

3. Turn your right foot out 90° and your left foot in slightly. Bend your right knee to form a right angle. Keep your left leg poker stiff.

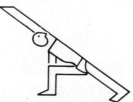

4. Place your right finger tips or your palm on the floor behind your knee. Stretch your left arm over the ear, the palm facing down. This is *Utthita Parshva-kona-asana.*

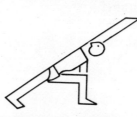

5. Come up. Return to position 2. Now turn your left foot out and your right foot in. Do the pose on the left side.

BENEFITS

✿ Strengthens leg muscles and joints

✿ Builds up stamina, good for athletes.

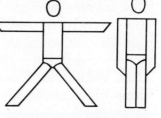

6. Come up. Return to position 2. Then jump back to Tada-asana.

DO

○ Turn your waist and broaden your chest.

○ Keep your elbows straight.

DON'T

☐ Don't project your buttocks backwards or bring your bent-knee forward.

9. Parivritta Parshva-kona-asana

10 to 20 counts each side

Parivritta means twisted or revolved, parshva means side, and kona means an angle. This is the twisted side angle pose. While twisting you form a spiral. Creepers climb in spirals. Seashells grow in spirals. In fact, many scientists believe that the entire universe is evolving in a spiral form.

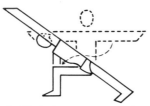

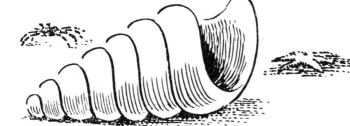

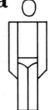

1. Stand in Tada-asana.

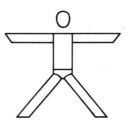

2. Jump and spread your legs 3 to 4 feet apart and your arms sideways, stand on a line, toes pointing forward and palms turned down.

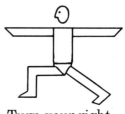

3. Turn your right foot out 90° and your left foot in 45°. Bend your right knee to form a right angle. Keep your left leg poker stiff.

4. Rotate your waist and fix your left shoulder behind your right knee. Place your left fingertips or palm on the floor. Stretch your right arm over the ear. Look up at your fingertips. This is *Parivritta Parshva-kona-asana*.

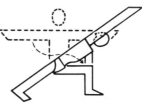

5. Come up. Return to position 2. Now turn your left foot out and your right foot in. Do the pose on the left side.

BENEFITS

✿ Makes the spine supple and relieves backaches.

✿ Helps relieve constipation.

✿ Trims waist and hips.

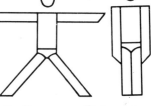

6. Come up. Return to position 2. Then jump back to Tada-asana.

DO

○ Remember, twists are contortions which remove distortions.

○ Raise the heel of your back leg if needed.

DON'T

☐ Don't bring your head forward.

10. Virabhadra-asana I

10 to 20 counts each side

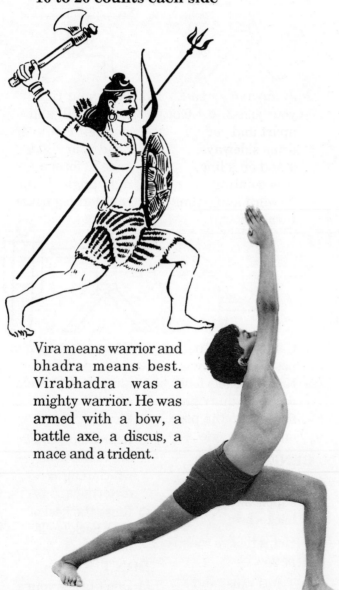

Vira means warrior and bhadra means best. Virabhadra was a mighty warrior. He was **armed** with a bow, a battle axe, a discus, a mace and a trident.

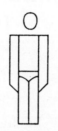

1. Stand in Tada-asana.

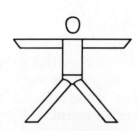

2. Jump and spread your legs 3 to 4 feet apart and your arms sideways. Stand on a line, toes pointing forward and palms turned down.

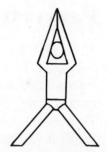

3. Turn the palms up. Raise your arms. Keep your elbows straight.

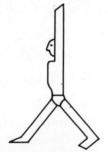

4. Turn **your right** foot out 90° and your left foot in 45° Revolve your hips and turn your trunk to the right.

DO

○ Be firm and strong like a warrior.

DON'T

☐ Don't lean forward.

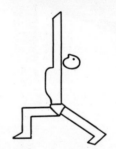

5. Bend **your** knee to form a right angle. Keep your left leg poker stiff. Look up at your fingertips. This is *Virabhadra-asana I.*

BENEFITS

✿ Increases stamina. Develops the lungs and chest

✿ Strengthens the shoulders and the back muscles.

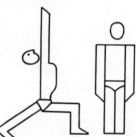

6. Come up. Return to position 3. **Do the** pose on the **left** side. Again come up, return to position 3, and jump back to Tada-asana.

11. Virabhadra-asana II

10 to 20 counts each side

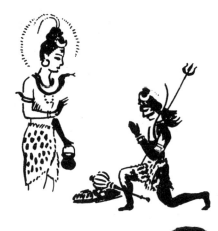

After destroying Daksha's sacrifice, Virabhadra the ferocious warrior, continued to rampage. To calm him, Lord Shiva granted him a boon. "You shall one day become a planet in the sky called Mangla (Mars). Many people shall worship you." So to this day many people in India worship the planet Mars.

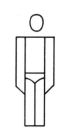

1. Stand in Tada-asana.

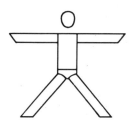

2. Jump and spread your legs 3 to 4 feet apart and your arms sideways. Stand on a line, toes pointing forward and palms turned down.

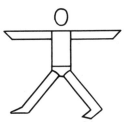

3. Turn your right foot out 90° and your left foot in slightly.

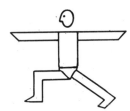

4. Bend your right knee to form a right angle. Keep your left leg poker stiff. Look at your right fingertips. This is *Virabhadra-asana II.*

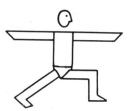

5. Come up. Return to position 2. Now turn your left foot out and your right foot in. Do the pose on the left side.

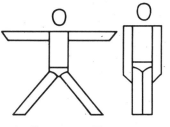

6. Come up. Return to position 2. Then jump back to Tada-asana.

DO
○ Stretch your arms as if you are being pulled apart in opposite directions.
○ Lift your **stomach up** and expand your chest.

DON'T
☐ Don't lean forward or sideways.

BENEFITS
✿ Makes legs powerful.
✿ Strengthens the back and stomach muscles.

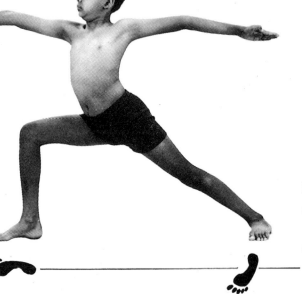

12. Virabhadra-asana III

10 to 20 counts each side

In olden times demons often harrased the gods and sages. So Virabhadra used his might to defend them.

Once, a demon snake swallowed many gods. Virabhadra slaughtered the snake and saved the gods.

Another time, several great sages were burnt by a raging fire. Virabhadra swallowed the fire. Then he used his magic powers to bring the sages back to life.

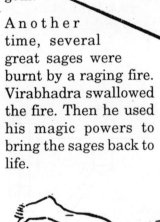

On a third occasion, a great demon swallowed many gods and sages. After a terrible battle Virabhadra defeated the demon and once again save the gods. Delighted at his courage and nobility Lord Shiva granted Virabhadra many boons.

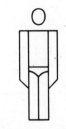

1. Stand in Tada-asana.

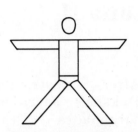

2. Jump and spread your legs 3 to 4 feet apart and your arms sideways. Stand on a line, toes pointing forward and palms turned down.

3. Then turn the palms up. Raise your arms. Tighten your elbows.

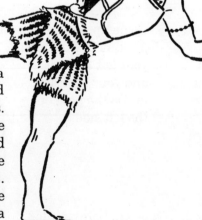

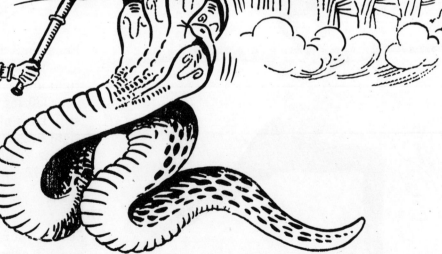

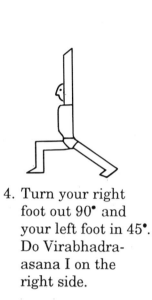 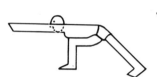 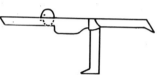 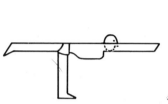 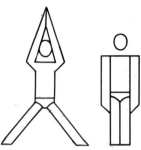

4. Turn your right foot out 90° and your left foot in 45°. Do Virabhadra-asana I on the right side.

5. Rest your chest on your thigh. Stretch your arms forward.

6. Raise your left leg off the floor. Straighten your right leg and balance on it. This is Vira-bhadra asana-III

7. Return to Virabhadra-asana I. Then come to position 3. Proceed step-by-step and perform the pose on the left side.

8. Return again to Virabhadra-asana I. Then come to position 3. Finally, jump back to Tada-asana.

DO

 Form a capital `T'.

○ Imagine your fingers are arrows shooting forward.

DON'T

□ Don't bend your knees or elbows.

□ Don't move the foot on which your are standing.

BENEFITS

 Improves balance and concentration.

✿ Builds strength and stamina.

13. Ardha Chandra-asana

10 to 20 counts each side

Ardha means half and Chandra means moon. Chandra was born when the sea was churned by the gods and the demons, (see Kurma-asana). When Chandra came of age, he married the twenty seven lunar constellations, who were Daksha's daughters.

One day the daughters complained to their father, "Our husband loves only our sister, Rohini. He neglects the rest of us."

In a fit of rage Daksha cursed the moon: "Chandra," said Daksha, "you will fade away and die."

Horrified, Chandra's wives begged their father to withdraw such a terrible curse. It was not possible to withdraw the curse. Daksha, however, agreed to change it. "Chandra, you will henceforth fade for a fortnight and grow for a fortnight."

That is why the moon continuously waxes and wanes.

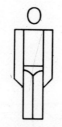

1. Stand in Tada-asana.

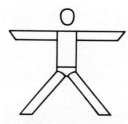

2. Jump and spread your legs 2 to 3 feet apart and your arms sideways. Stand on a line, toes pointing forward and palms turned down.

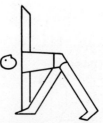

3. Turn your right foot out 90° and your left foot in slightly. Do Utthita Trikona-asana on the right side.

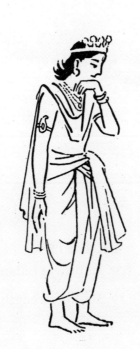

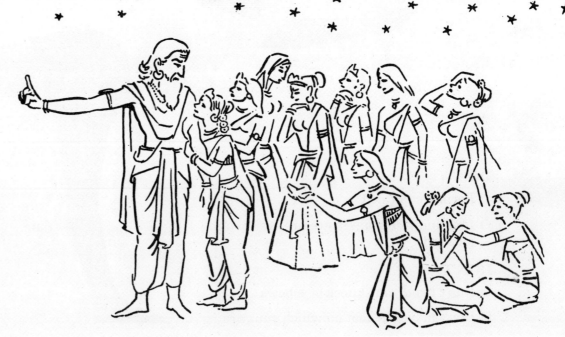

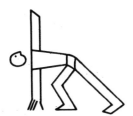

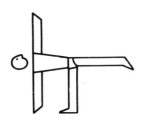

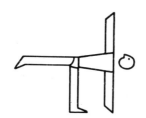

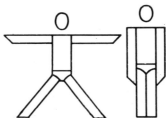

4. Bend your right knee. Place your right fingertips in front of your right foot.

5. Raise your left leg off the floor. Straighten your right leg and balance. Look up at your fingertips. This is *Ardha Chandra-asana.*

6. Return to Utthita Trikona-asana. Come up. Now turn your left foot out and the right foot in. Do Ardha Chandra- asana on the left side, step-by-step.

7. Return to Utthita Trikona-asana. Come up. Return to position 2. Then jump back to Tada-asana.

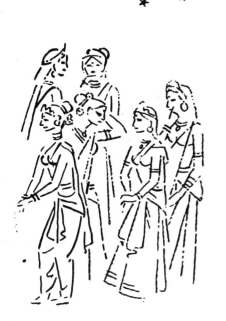

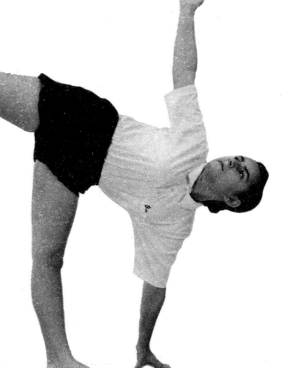

DO

○ Rotate your chest towards the ceiling.

DON'T

□ Don't shift the foot on which you are standing.

□ Don't let your head hang down or bring the head forward.

BENEFITS

✿ Develops the legs correctly.

✿ Strengthens the lower back and pelvic region.

14. Parshva-uttana-asana

15 to 20 counts each side

Parshva means side, and uttana means intense pull. Parshva-uttana-asana stretches the sides of the legs and trunk.

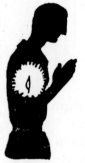 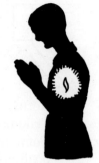

Indians traditionally greet people with palms folded in front of the chest—*namaste*. Namaste means 'I bow to the Light within you'. In Parshva-uttana asana the *namaste* is performed with the palms folded behind one's own back. The yogi here bows to the light that dwells within himself. This light which dwells within each of us has many names: atma, soul, spirit, God.

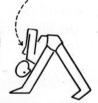

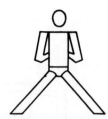

1. Stand in Tada-asana.

2. Fold your palms behind your back, *namaste*. Jump and spread your legs 2 to 3 feet apart. Stand on a line. Toes pointing forward.

3. Turn your right foot out 90° and your left foot 45° in. Turn your trunk to the right. Throw your head back.

Bend forward. Bring your head to your right knee. This is *Parshva-uttana-asana*.

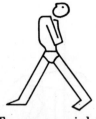

5. Come up. Return to position 2. Now turn your left foot out and your right foot in. Do the pose on the left side.

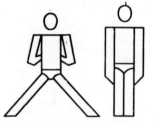

6. Come up. Return to position 2. Then jump back to Tada-asana.

DO

○ Tighten your knees and your thigh muscles.

○ Draw your shoulder back. Press the palms against each other.

DON'T

☐ Don't bring your knee to your head, instead bring your head to your knee.

BENEFITS

✿ Corrects round shoulders.

✿ Makes the hip joints flexible.

✿ Expands the lungs, develops the chest.

15. Prasarita Pada-uttana-asana

15 to 20 seconds

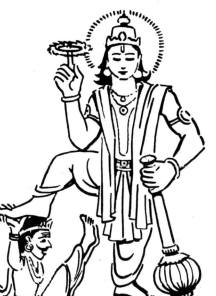

Prasarita means spread. Pada means leg. Uttana means intense. Once there was a wicked and powerful king named Bali. To rid the world of this menace, the gods prayed to Lord Vishnu. In answer to their prayers Vishnu was born as a dwarf, Vamana.

Though wicked, Bali was renowned for his generosity. One day the dwarf Vamana went to Bali and sought a boon of him. "O King! grant me as much land as I can cover with three steps, said the dwarf." Laughing, Bali granted him his wish.

Instantly, the dwarf grew very tall. With one wide step he crossed the earth. With a second great step he crossed the heavens. For the third step Vamana had nowhere to place his foot. So he stepped on Bali's head and pushed him into the underworld.

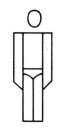

1. Stand in Tada-asana.

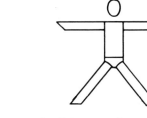

2. Jump and spread your legs 3 to 4 feet apart. Stand on a line, toes pointing forward.

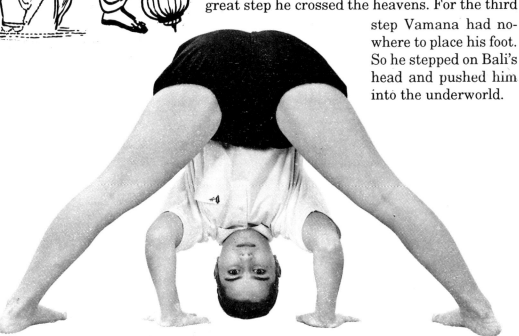

3. Place your palms on the floor, fingers pointing forward. Look up.

DO

○ Keep your feet, palms and head all in one line.

DON'T

☐ Don't bend your knees.

☐ Don't turn your toes out.

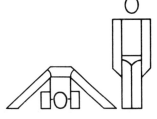

4. Rest the crown of your head on the floor. This is *Prasarita Pada-uttana-asana.* Then raise your head. Jump back to Tada-asana.

BENEFITS

✿ Removes fatigue

✿ Improves arches

✿ Relieves cramps in the calves.

The Sun-Salutation Poses

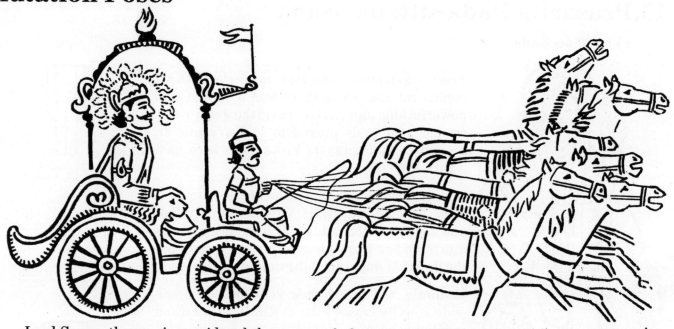

Lord Surya, the sun, is considered the source of light, heat and knowledge. He rides across the sky in a chariot pulled by seven shining horses. Once, Hanuman, the monkey god, approached Lord Surya and bowed low before him. "O Lord," he prayed, "please accept me as your humble student so that I may grow in knowledge and wisdom." The sun agreed, "I accept you as my student, but you may not sit in my chariot. You must walk before the chariot studying the scriptures."

Surya Namaskar

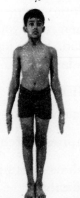
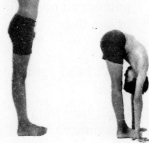
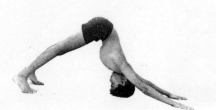
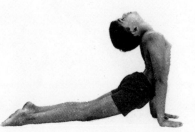

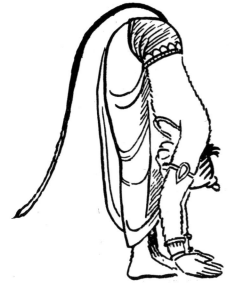

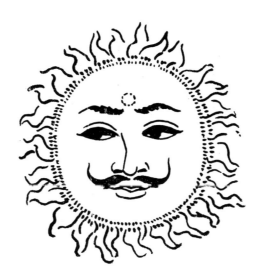

Hanuman accepted the challenge. With his book open in his hand, Hanuman crossed the skies walking in front of Surya's chariot. Very soon he mastered all the scriptures and became a wise and learned monkey.

The yogis, too, invoke the blessings of the sun. To do this they perform a sequence of bending and bowing movements called the Sun-Salutation Poses or Surya Namaskar. These asanas are performed in quick succession, often jumping from pose to pose. The entire sequence is repeated several times.

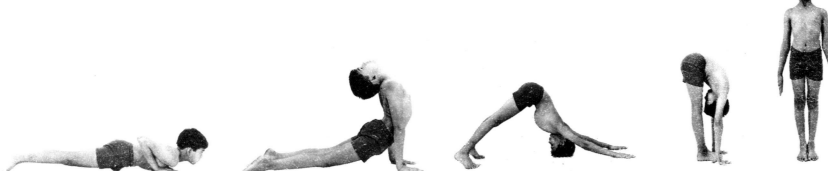

16. Uttana-asana

20 to 100 counts

Ut means intensely and tana means to stretch. There once grew a huge oak tree. Beside the tree grew a bamboo thicket. Every day the oak boasted "I am the tallest, the strongest and the hardest tree around." One day the wind god heard the boast. That evening he created a wild storm.

The hard and rigid oak was unable to bend with the wind and so it was uprooted. The supple bamboo just bent to the wind's might.

We must also learn to keep ourselves strong and supple like the bamboo. Then we can weather the storms of life.

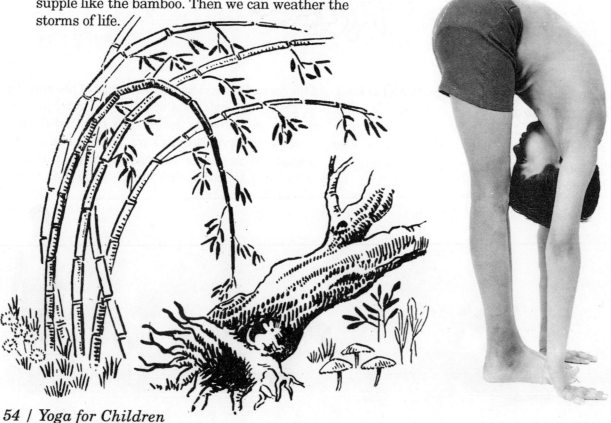

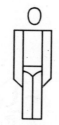

1. Stand in Tada-asana.

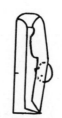

2. Bend forward. Touch your toes. Pull up your knee-caps. Tighten your thighs.

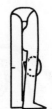

3. Bend further. Hold your ankles or place your hands by the sides of your feet. Touch your head to your knee. This is *Uttana-asana*.

DO

○ Let your head hang loose.

DON'T

☐ Don't let your knees buckle.

☐ Don't stiffen your neck.

BENEFITS

✿ Removes fatigue.

✿ Exercises the organs: stomach, liver, kidneys, heart.

✿ Improves concentration.

17. Chatur-anga Danda-asana

5 to 10 seconds

Chatur means four and anga means limbs. Danda means a rod, it also means to prostrate. To show respect Indians often go down on all four limbs, or even stretch themselves fully on the ground.

Upon completing his studies, Hanuman approached his guru, the sun. "O, Guru" he said, "please accept a gift from your humble student."

"I am satisfied with your efforts," replied the sun god. "I require no other gift."

Hanuman insisted that his teacher accept a gift. Surya consented. "Go to the earth," said Lord Surya, "and serve my son, the monkey king Sugriva." Happily Hanuman went to the earth and served as Sugriva's loyal minister for many years.

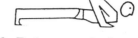

1. Lie on your stomach. Place your palms beside your chest. The fingers pointing forward.

2. Raise your body slightly off the floor, like a push-up. Remain parallel to the floor. This is *Chatur-anga Danda-asana*.

DO

○ Be straight as a rod.

DON'T

☐ Don't let your buttocks protrude

BENEFITS

✿ Strengthens muscles of the arms and shoulders.

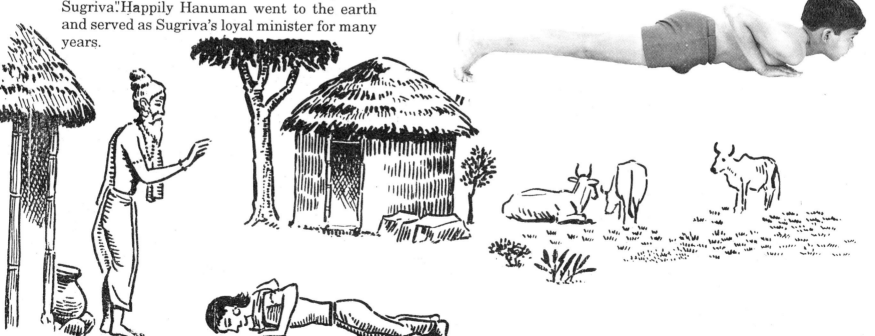

18. Adho Mukha Shvana-asana

30 to 60 counts

Adho means down and mukha means face. Shvana means dog. Have you seen a dog stretch? This pose resembles a dog stretching its front legs. Remember, stretching refreshes a dog, so stretch well.

BENEFITS

✿ Tones the leg muscles, good for runners.

✿ Removes fatigue.

✿ Refreshes a tired brain.

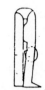
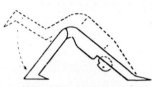
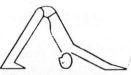

1. Stand in Uttana-asana. Rest your palms on the floor.

DO

○ Stretch like a dog, dip in your back.

DON'T

☐ Don't make your back round like a cat.

☐ Don't turn your toes out.

☐ Don't bend your knees and elbows.

2. Take a big step back or jump back. Keep your feet about 12 inches apart. Let the fingers and toes be well spread and pointing forward.

3. Form an inverted 'V' shape. Stretch your arms and legs. Bring your head to the floor. This is *Adho Mukha Shvana-asana*.

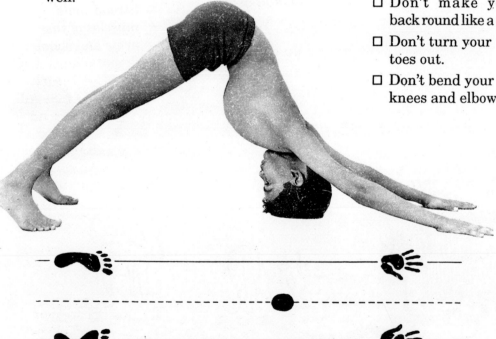

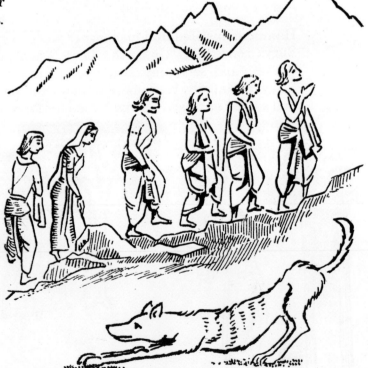

19. Urdhva Mukha Shvana-asana

10 to 20 counts

Urdhva means upwards and mukha means face. Shvana means dog. This pose resembles a dog stretching its hind legs. In the epic *Mahabharata*, it is told that after winning the great battle, the five Pandava brothers ruled for 36 years. Feeling old age approaching, they handed the kingdom to their successors. Then the brothers and their wife Draupadi set out for the high Himalayas. A lean and hungry dog joined them on the way. First Draupadi collapsed of exhaution. Then four of the Pandava brothers also fell along the way. Only the eldest brother, the virtuous Yudhishthira accompanied by the faithful dog, reached the high Himalayas.

Lord Indra arrived in his chariot and invited Yudhishthira to heaven. Seeing his faithful dog wagging its tail, Yudhishthira stepped aside to let it enter the chariot first. "This dirty dog cannot come to heaven", shouted Indra

"He is my loyal companion," said Yudhishthira. "If he may not join me then I, too, shall not come to heaven."

Delighted at hearing these words, the dog assumed its true form. The dog was none other than Yama, the god of justice. Yama had put Yudhishthira to one last test.

Indra then took Yudhishthira to heaven.

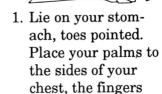

1. Lie on your stomach, toes pointed. Place your palms to the sides of your chest, the fingers pointing forward.

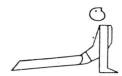

2. Straighten your arms. Raise your thighs and trunk off the floor. Thrust your chest forward. Throw your head back. This is *Urdhva Mukha Shvana-asana.*

DO

○ Tuck in your tailbone.

○ Draw your shoulders back.

DON'T

☐ Don't bend your knees and elbows.

BENEFITS

✡ Makes the spine strong and supple.

The Inverted Poses

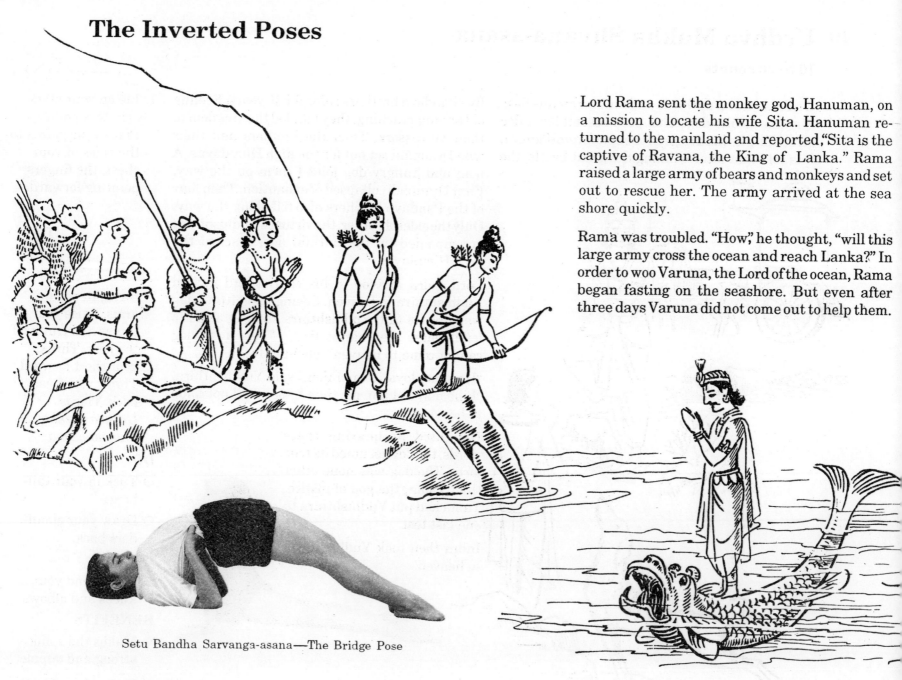

Lord Rama sent the monkey god, Hanuman, on a mission to locate his wife Sita. Hanuman returned to the mainland and reported, "Sita is the captive of Ravana, the King of Lanka." Rama raised a large army of bears and monkeys and set out to rescue her. The army arrived at the sea shore quickly.

Rama was troubled. "How," he thought, "will this large army cross the ocean and reach Lanka?" In order to woo Varuna, the Lord of the ocean, Rama began fasting on the seashore. But even after three days Varuna did not come out to help them.

Setu Bandha Sarvanga-asana—The Bridge Pose

Enraged at Varuna's pride, Rama unleashed a fiery arrow deep into the waters. Varuna hastily appeared and bowed before Lord Rama with folded palms: "I will guide your army where to build a bridge. I shall also bear the boulders and trees your soldiers throw into the waters so that your bridge may be firm." Varuna then returned to the depths of ocean.

The bears and monkeys set to work without delay. Jambavan, the king of the bears, Sugriva, the king of the monkeys, and Nala and Hanuman, Sugriva's ministers spurred them on. They dug up great boulders and hurled them into the ocean, "Splash!" Great trees were uprooted and dropped in. The top of the path was made smooth with mud and small pieces of wood. Speedily, the sea was bridged. Rama's army swiftly crossed the ocean to wage war against Ravana, the wicked king of Lanka.

Ever since those days this "bridge" has been called Setu Bandha.

20. Shirsha-asana

1 to 3 minutes

Shirsha means head. This is the head-stand. Ravana's mother was a great devotee of Lord Shiva. One day someone stole the Linga, the symbol of Lord Shiva, which she used for worship. Seeing his mother's grief, Ravana consoled her, "I will bring you a Linga from Shiva himself."

Ravana then set off for the high Himalayas to do penance. There he lit five big fires. In the centre, with fires blazing around him, Ravana stood on his head for ten thousand years.

Pleased by Ravana's efforts, Lord Shiva appeared before him and offered him three boons. Ravana asked, "Make me immortal, give me your wife Parvati for a bride, and give me a Linga." Although he was annoyed, Lord Shiva granted these wishes.

Happily Ravana set off homewards. Along the way he met the mischievious sage, Narada. "How can you be made immortal?" scoffed Narada. "This is impossible." Thinking that he had been tricked, Ravana returned to Shiva's abode and disturbed Shiva's meditation. Promptly Shiva withdrew the gift of immortality.

Sadly Ravana walked on. Then the gods played a trick on him. They made Parvati appear as an old hag. Ravana rejected her, and so lost his second boon.

Carrying his precious Linga, Ravana journeyed on. Tired, he halted a while to rest and placed the Linga on the ground. The Linga sank deep into the earth.

The proud king Ravana lost all the boons he had obtained through his efforts.

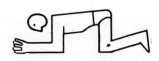

1. Kneel in front of a folded blanket. Rest your forearms on the blanket. Firmly interlock your fingers. Form a cup-shape with your palms.

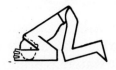

2. Place the crown of your head on the blanket. Allow the back of your head to fit into your cupped palms.

3. Raise your knees off the floor. Take 2 or 3 little steps towards your head.

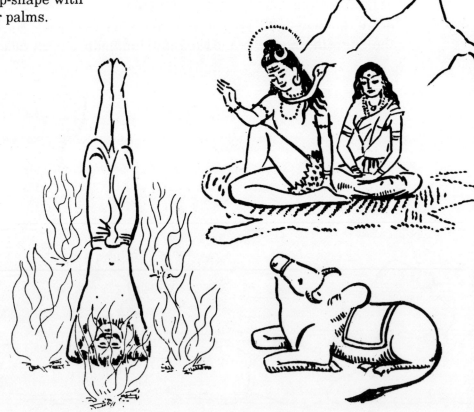

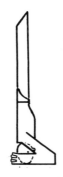 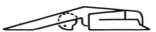

4. Lift your feet off the ground! Move upwards with flexed knees.

5. Then straighten your legs. Keep your inverted body perpendicular to the floor. Join your legs. Keep them poker stiff. Point your toes. This is *Shirsha-asana.*

6. Then come down. Land on your toes. Remain with your head down (as in Virasana III) for 10 to 15 seconds.

DO

○ Learn the pose by taking the support of a wall. Keep only your knuckles and heels touching the wall.

○ Fall correctly when learning to balance without support. Simply loosen your fingers and roll onto your back.

○ Always lift your shoulders and broaden your chest.

DON'T

☐ Don't widen your elbows more than the width of your shoulders.

☐ Don't rest on your forehead or on the back of your head, nor tilt your head to a side.

☐ Don't throw your legs backwards or forward, nor lean them to a side.

BENEFITS

✿ Increases blood circulation in the brain.

✿ Improves concentration, memory and will power.

✿ Promotes growth.

✿ Removes fatigue, builds up energy.

✿ Strengthens the entire body, increases resistance to sickness.

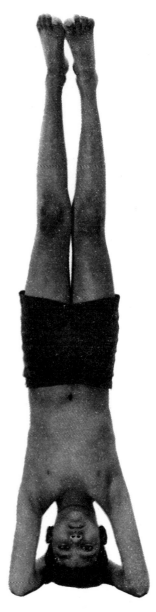

Yoga for Children / 61

21. Sarvanga-asana

1 to 3 minutes

Sarva means all and anga means parts. In shape Sarvanga-asana resembles a popular Indian musical instrument, the tambura. The tambura is a stringed instrument with a sweet sound. It is the favourite instrument of Sage Narada, the chief musician of the gods.

The tambura is an instrument used for intoning. Sarvanga-asana too, helps tone all parts of the body. This pose also soothes the mind and emotions bringing the body and mind in harmony.

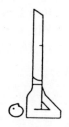

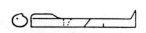
1. Lie on your back.

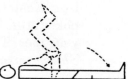
2. Bend your knees towards your chest. Raise your hips and legs off the floor. Support your back with your palms.

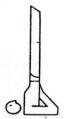
3. Straighten your legs. Be perpendicular to the floor. Let only the back of your head, neck, shoulders and upper-arms touch the floor.

4. Join and tighten your legs. Point your toes. This is *Sarvanga-asana*.

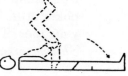
5. Then bend your knees and come down gently.

DO
○ Tuck in your tail-bone.
○ Press your palms into the back of the chest and raise your spine upwards.

DON'T
□ Don't place your elbows wider than your shoulders.
□ Don't tilt your head.
□ Don't bring your legs forward.

BENEFITS
✿ Promotes **growth** and health.
✿ Helps relieve headaches, colds, coughs constipation.
✿ Refreshes the body, soothes the nerves.
✿ Improves functioning of vital organs, glands and nerves.

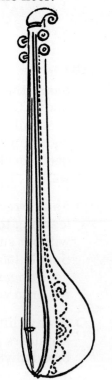

22. Hala-asana

1 to 2 minutes

23. Karna-pida-asana

30 to 60 counts

Hala means plough. A long, long time ago there lived a wise king named Janaka. He had everything a king could wish for but great as he was, he had no children.

To seek the blessings of the gods, Janaka decided to conduct a religious ceremony. He started ploughing the earth to prepare the ceremonial spot. During the ploughing a shining golden box was discovered. Inside it Janaka found a beautiful baby girl. He took her home and named her, Sita, which means furrow.

To celebrate his earth-born child he put the symbol of a plough on his royal banner. Thereafter he was called the King-with-the-Plough-Banner.

Karna means ear and pida means pressure. In this pose you put pressure on the ears with your knees.

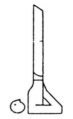

1. Do Sarvanga-asana.

DO

○ Keep your back and your legs straight and stiff as a plough.

BENEFITS

✿ Keeps the spine supple and healthy.

✿ Helps relieve digestive problems.

✿ Rests the brain and make you calm and quiet.

2. Bring your legs down over your head. Rest your toes on the floor. Keep your legs poker stiff. This is *Hala-asana*.

DON'T

☐ Don't tumble to a side.

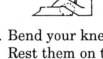

3. Bend your knees. Rest them on the floor beside your ears. Rest your arms on your calves. Point your toes. This is *Karna-pida-asana*.

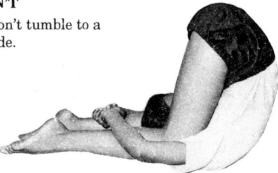

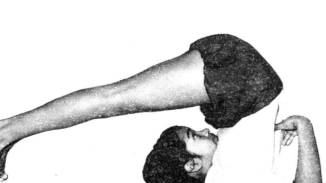

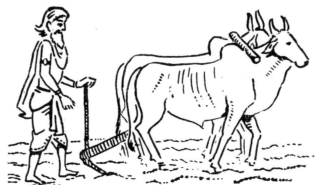

24. Setu Bandha Sarvanga-asana

1 to 2 minutes

This pose is a variation of Sarvanga-asana.

Setu means bridge and bandha means construction or formation. Setu bandha is the name of the bridge which the bears and monkeys are said to have built for Rama. It extended across the sea from the coast of south-east India to Sri Lanka. Today all that is left of the bridge is a ridge of rocks in the ocean. On maps it is called Adam's Bridge.

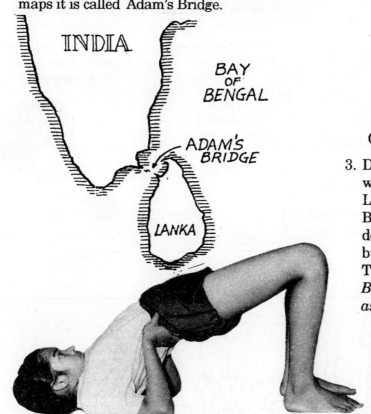

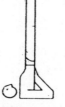

1. Do Sarvanga-asana.

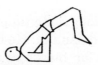

2. Bend your knees backwards. Bring your elbows nearer each other. Tighten your buttocks. Arch your back.

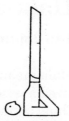

5. Then return to Sarvanga-asana **and lie flat on your back.**

3. Drop backwards with bent knees. Land on your toes. Bring your heels down. Keep your buttocks raised. This is *Setu Bandha Sarvanga-asana.* (easy pose).

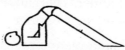

4. Slowly straighten your legs. Join your feet and knees. Tighten your buttocks. This is *Setu Bandha Sarvanga-asana* (final pose).

DO
○ Always place your palms and wrists as in Sarvanga-asana.

DON'T
☐ **Don't raise your shoulders off the floor.**
☐ **Don't collapse your bridge by sagging at the centre.**

BENEFITS
✿ Strengthens the wrists.
✿ Tones up the kidneys.
✿ Makes the spine strong and healthy.
✿ Improves breathing.
✿ Refreshes the body and mind.

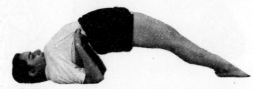

25. Adho Mukha Vriksha-asana

20 to 40 counts

Adho means down, mukha means face and vriksha means tree. This is the upside down tree pose. What could have inspired this pose?

The peculiar banyan tree perhaps? The banyan is a common Indian tree. Some of it's branches grow downwards instead of growing upwards. The ends of these branches grow into the soil and become roots. Over time, a single banyan tree could become a whole grove.

The banyan is a sacred tree. In India many trees and plants are considered sacred. Sages had great respect for trees. A sage once said, "If you plant even one tree you go to heaven."

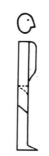

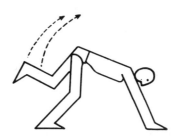

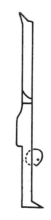

1. Stand in Tada-asana.

2. Bend down. Place your palms on the floor, fingers well spread and pointing forward. Keep your arms straight.

3. Swing your legs upwards. Balance as in hand-stand, toes pointed. This is *Adho Mukha Vriksha-asana.*

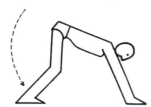

4. Then come down. Land on your toes.

DO

○ Lean against a wall. Keep your finger tips about 4" away from the wall.

○ Stretch up.

DON'T

☐ Don't bend your elbows.

BENEFITS

✿ Strengthens the wrists, arms, shoulders.

✿ Makes the mind alert.

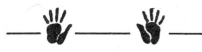

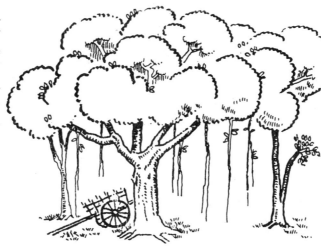

The Cross-Legged Poses

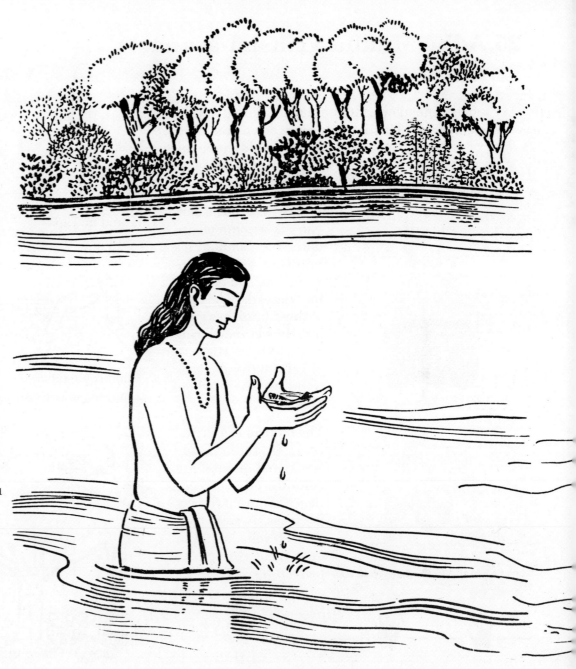

There once lived a wise king named Manu. One day while Manu was bathing in the river, a little fish sought shelter in his cupped palms. "Save me," it said, "and some day I shall help you."

Amazed, Manu placed the fish in a pot of water. Overnight the fish outgrew the pot. So Manu placed it in a well. Very shortly it grew too large to live in the well. Astonished, Manu placed this magic fish in a large lake. Sure enough, it soon outgrew the lake. So Manu led it the river, Ganga. The fish continued to grow. Manu now realised that this fish could be none other than the great Lord Vishnu. Reverentially, he took it to the ocean.

Pleased with Manu's dedication and devotion, the fish confirmed that it was, indeed, a form of Lord Vishnu. It warned Manu of an approaching flood which would drown the whole earth. It instructed him to build a ship, and to load it with the eggs and the young of plants, insects, birds, mammals and all other living creatures. Manu wisely followed the divine counsel.

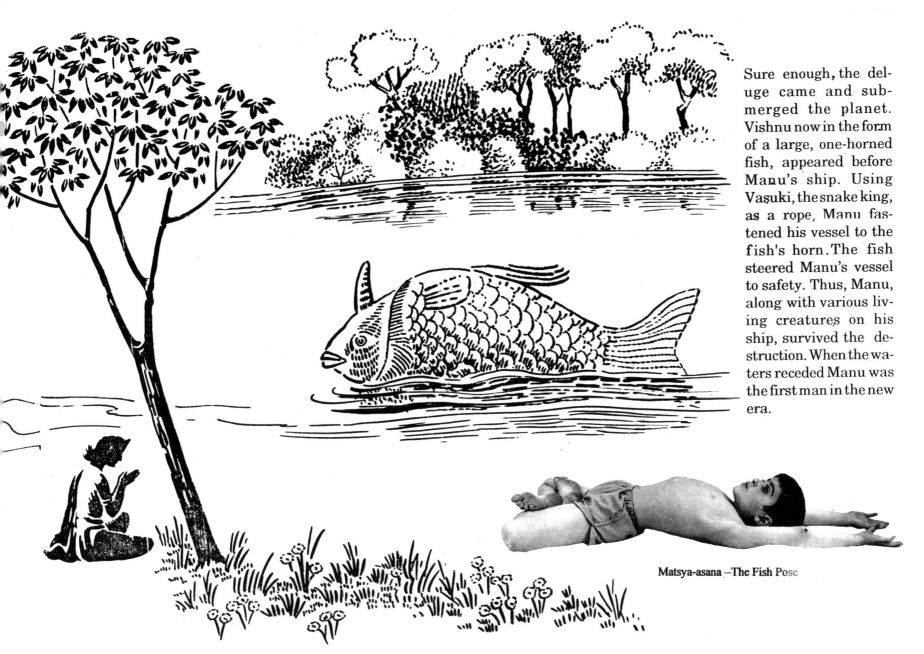

Sure enough, the deluge came and submerged the planet. Vishnu now in the form of a large, one-horned fish, appeared before Manu's ship. Using Vasuki, the snake king, as a rope, Manu fastened his vessel to the fish's horn. The fish steered Manu's vessel to safety. Thus, Manu, along with various living creatures on his ship, survived the destruction. When the waters receded Manu was the first man in the new era.

Matsya-asana —The Fish Pose

26. Padma-asana

30 to 60 counts each side

Padma means lotus. The lotus is a symbol of purity. Lotus seeds sprout in the dark, murky bottom of a pond. The lotus stems grow upwards towards the light of the sun. Above the surface of the pond, unspoilt by the muddy waters, the beautiful lotus flowers bloom.

We too should try and be pure like the lotus. Keep away from the muddy waters of bad thoughts and deeds.

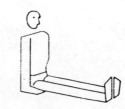

1. Sit in Dandasana.

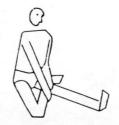

2. Bend your right knee. Hold your right ankle and the foot. Place it at the root of your left thigh.

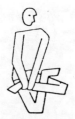

3. Then bend your left knee. Hold your left ankle and foot and place it at the root of your right thigh.

4. Rest the back of your palms on your knees. Perform the Jnana Mudra by joining the tips of the thumbs with the index fingers. Sit erect.

5. Then return to Danda-asana. Repeat the pose crossing your legs the other way, first bend the left knee and then the right knee. This is *Padma-asana*.

DO

○ Make a compact Padma-asana. Bring your knees closer together. Press them to the floor.

DON'T

☐ Don't slouch.

BENEFITS

✿ Teaches you to sit correctly with the back straight.

✿ Refreshes the body and makes the mind alert.

✿ Keeps the knee, hip and ankle joints strong and flexible.

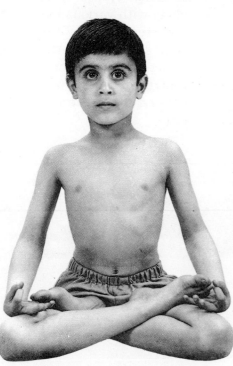

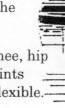
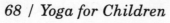

27. Matsya-asana

1 to 2 minutes each side

Matsya means fish. Once while Lord Brahma, the creator, was reciting the scriptures, (the Vedas) a crafty demon crept up and stole them. He dived into the depths of the ocean and hid there with the scriptures. To retrieve the sacred books Lord Vishnu changed himself into a fish. The fish defeated the demon and recovered the scriptures. This divine fish also saved Manu from the great flood.

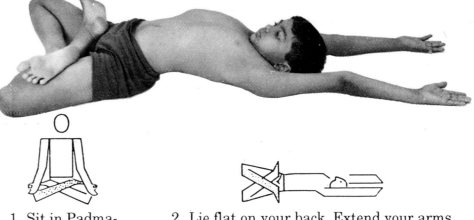

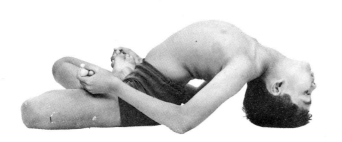

1. Sit in Padma-asana.

2. Lie flat on your back. Extend your arms overhead. Lengthen your spine. This is *Matsya-asana*.

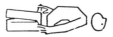

3. Now hook both your big toes with your index and middle fingers. Place your elbows on the floor. Arch your back and rest the crown of your head on the floor. This is *Matsya-asana II*.

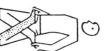

4. Then change the crossing of your legs. Repeat positions 2 and 3. Finally sit up in Padma-asana.

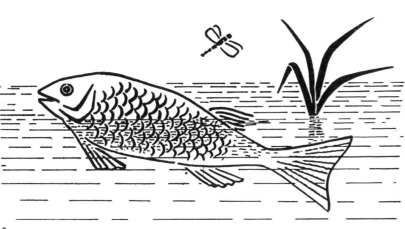

DO

○ Imagine you are a fish. Your folded legs are your tail and your bent elbows are your fins.

○ Press your thighs and knees to the floor.

DON'T

□ Don't loosen your crossed-legs.

BENEFITS

✡ Refreshes the body and mind.

✡ Keeps the abdominal organs healthy.

28. Parvata-asana

20 to 30 counts each side

Parvata means mountain. A long, long time ago all mountains had wings. They flew about swiftly and landed where they pleased. Naturally, men and beasts lived in great fear of a big mountain crashing down on their heads at any moment.

Some pious sages complained to Lord Indra, "Please help us, O Lord. Rid the world of this menace of flying mountains."

Lord Indra requested the mountains to remain in one place. The mountains refused. Enraged, Indra chopped off their wings with his thunder bolt. Ever since then mountains remain steady and rooted in one place.

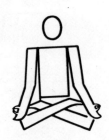

1. Sit in Padma-asana.

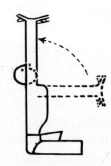

2. Interlock your fingers. Turn the palms out. Extend your arms forward. Then raise your arms overhead. This is *Parvata-asana*.

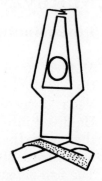

3. Bring your arms down. Uncross your legs and recross them the other way. Repeat the pose.

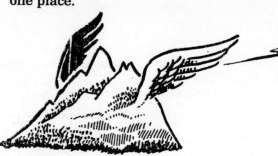

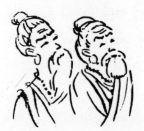

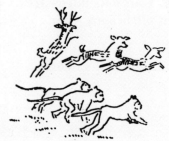

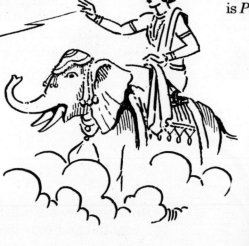

DO

- Lift your shoulder blades upwards.
- Keep your raised arms behind your ears.

DON'T

- Don't bend your elbows.

BENEFITS

- Corrects a rounded back and drooping shoulders.
- Makes wrists flexible.

29. Tola-asana

5 to 10 counts

Tola means a pair of scales. This pose resembles one pan of a scale. Tola is also the zodiac constellation of Libra, the symbol of which is a pair of scales.

The Indian sages minutely observed the star spangled night skies. No less than six asanas can be related to zodiac constellations: Simha, Tola, Vrischika, Dhanur, Makara and Matsya, (Leo, Libra, Scorpio, Sagittarius, Capricorn, and Pisces).

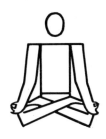

1. Sit in Padma-asana.

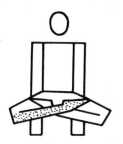

2. Place the palms on the floor besides your hips, fingers pointing forward. Raise your crossed-legs off the floor. Balance. This is *Tola-asana*.

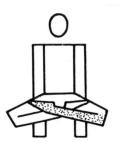

3. Then rest on the floor. Interchange the position of the legs and repeat the pose.

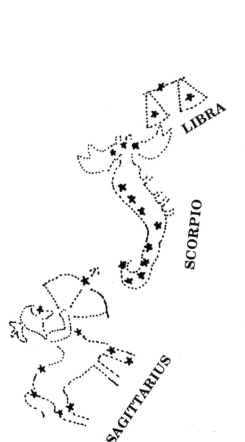

VIRGO

LIBRA

SCORPIO

SAGITTARIUS

LEO

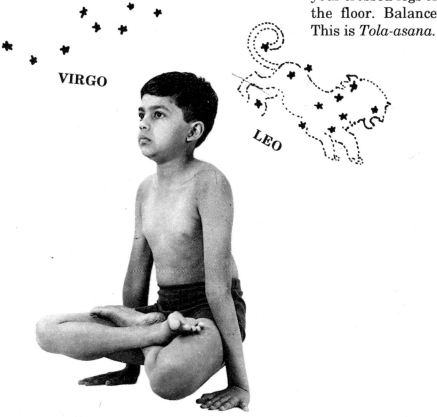

DO

○ Distribute your weight evenly on both palms.

○ Swing back and forth.

DON'T

☐ Don't look down.

BENEFITS

✿ Strengthens the fingers, wrists, arms and stomach muscles.

30. Simha-asana

10 to 20 counts

Simha means lion. There once lived a ferocious king named Hiranya-kashyapu. Through penance he had obtained the boon that he could neither be killed by man nor by beast, neither by day nor by night, neither while indoors nor when outdoors and neither by hand nor by weapon. Considering himself invincible, he wrecked havoc on earth.

Hiranya-kashyapu despised Lord Vishnu. Strangely enough Hiranya-kashyapu's son, Prahlada, was a pious boy and a great devotee of Vishnu. Hiranya-kashyapu tried to kill him, but each time Prahlada was protected by Lord Vishnu.

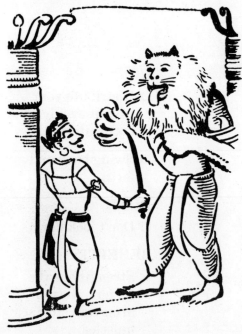

Finally Vishnu appeared in the form of a dreadful creature, half-man-half-lion, called Narasimha. It was twilight. The man-lion dragged Hiranya-kashyapu to the threshold. There, neither indoors, nor outdoors, Narasimha tore the evil king apart with his sharp claws.

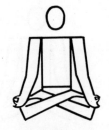

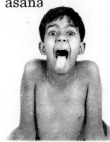

1. Sit in Padma-asana

4. Open your mouth wide. Stretch your tongue out towards your chin. Gaze at the tip of your nose or between the eyebrows. This is *Simha-asana*.

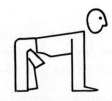

2. Place the palms on the floor in front of you, the fingers pointing forward. Raise your buttocks and come onto your hands and knees.

5. Then sit in Padma-asana. Interchange the crossing of the legs. Repeat the pose.

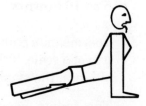

3. Move your buttocks down towards the floor. Keep your arms straight.

DO

○ Breathe loudly through your mouth.

○ Expand your chest.

DON'T

☐ Don't protrude your tail-bone.

BENEFITS

✿ Helps get rid of bad breath.

✿ Makes the lower spine elastic.

31. Goraksha-asana

4 to 5 counts

Go means cow and raksha means to protect. Go-raksha means cowherd. Little children are often cowherds. Even Lord Krishna, the most popular incarnation of Lord Vishnu, spent his childhood as a cowherd.

In Lord Krishna's time the villagers used to worship Lord Indra for rain. The cowherd Krishna opposed this. "Why, don't we worship Govardhana mountain, he said. It is the mountain which helps bring down the rain" he said. The villagers agreed. They stopped worshipping Lord Indra. "O Govardhana mountain", they prayed instead, "please send down the rain that makes the grass grow for our cattle."

1. Sit in Padma-asana.

2. Place your hands on the floor in front of you. Raise your buttocks off the floor.

3. Come onto your knees. Straighten your back and balance with folded palms. This is *Goraksha-asana*.

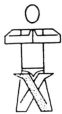

4. Return to the sitting position. Change the crossing of the legs. Repeat the pose.

DO

○ Tuck in your tailbone and tighten your buttocks.

DON'T

☐ Don't widen your knees.

BENEFITS

✿ A challenging and enjoyable pose.

✿ Brings mobility to the tail bone area, knee and ankle joints.

Angry, Indra hurled down thunderbolts, lightning and rain on the villagers. To protect his friends Lord Krishna lifted Govardhana mountain on his little finger. All the cowherds, villagers and their cattle sheltered under this huge umbrella.

The thunderstorm lasted seven days. Under Krishna's great umbrella the cowherds and their cattle remained safe and dry. At last Lord Indra accepted defeat. He came and bowed before Lord Krishna. Since that day Lord Krishna is affectionately called Govinda, Protector of Cows.

Several hundred years ago there was also a great yogi named Goraksha.

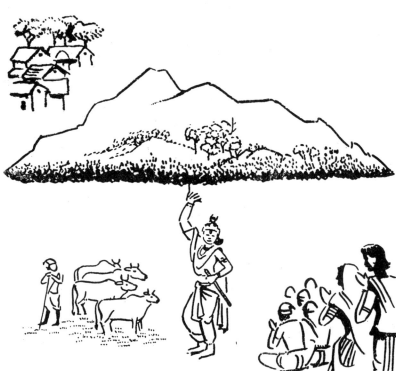

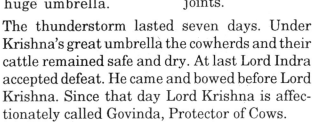

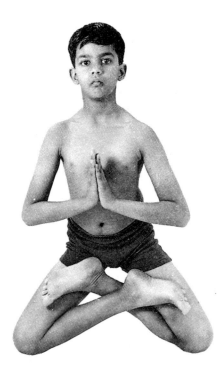

Yoga for Children / 73

32. Kukkuta-asana

5 to 10 counts

Kukkuta means a cock. A cock stands for good and correct judgement. It quickly picks out grain and small insects hidden or scattered in the soil.

Birds are very important in Indian legends. It is said that they know many secrets unknown to men. They are also the messengers of the gods. Several Indian gods ride on birds. The great Lord Vishnu rides on an eagle. Kama, the God of Love, rides on a parrot. Brahma, the creator, rides on a swan. Karttikeya, the war god, rides a peacock. He has a cock on his banner.

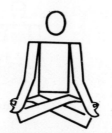

1. Sit in Padma-asana.

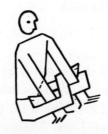

2. Insert your arms into the gaps between the calves and thighs. Push your arms in deeply.

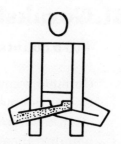

3. Place the palms on the floor with the fingers well spread. Raise your thighs and hips off the floor. Balance. This is *Kukkuta-asana*.

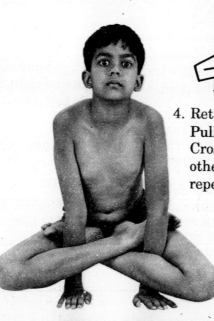

4. Return to the floor. Pull your arms out. Cross your legs the other way and repeat the pose.

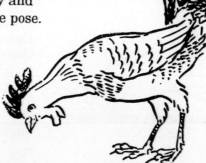

DO
○ Sway your trunk slightly forward in order to lift off.

DON'T
☐ Don't make the mistake of inserting your arms between the ankle and upper thigh.

BENEFITS
✿ Strengthens the fingers, wrists, arms and the muscles of the abdomen.

33. Baddha Padma-asana

20 to 30 counts

Baddha means tied or restrained and Padma-asana is the lotus-pose. Mudra means sealing or closing, and Yoga means joining. These poses are good examples of literally tying yourself in knots.

Why should one do this ? Because Yoga teaches mastery of one's own self and not of others. What does one have to master ? One's actions, speech, thoughts and feelings. Self discipline leads to wisdom.

A great sage was once asked, "Who is greater, the king or the sage?". The sage replied, "The king conquers others, the sage conquers himself. So the sage is greater."

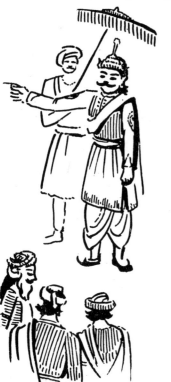

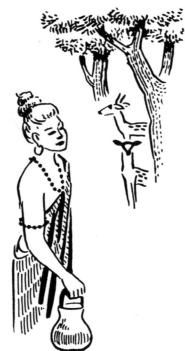

34. Yoga Mudra-asana

20 to 30 counts

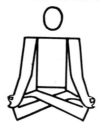

1. Sit in Padma-asana. Bend your right knee first and then the left.

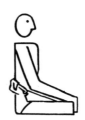

2. Breathe out sharply and throw your left arm behind your back. Catch hold of your left big toe.

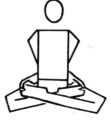

3. Then throw your right arm behind your back and catch hold of your right big toe. Look straight. This is *Baddha Padma-asana.*

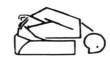

4. Bend forward. Rest your forehead on the ground. This is *Yoga-Mudra-asana.*

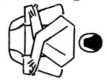

5. Then sit erect. Recross your legs and the arms. Repeat Baddha Padma-asana and Yoga Mudra-asana.

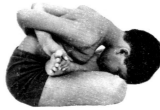

DO
- Cross your legs tightly. Squeeze your knees towards each other.

DON'T
- Don't get disheartened if you can't catch hold of your toes. Hold your T-shirt instead.

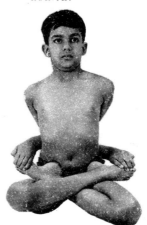

BENEFITS
- Improves respiration.
- Strengthens the shoulders, good for sportsmen.

The Forward Bending Poses

The gods were constantly losing battles against the demons. Worried, they sought Lord Vishnu's aid.

"Go and befriend the demons," advised Vishnu. "Take their help and churn the ocean for amrit, the nectar of immortality. Drink this nectar and you will become invincible."

The gods followed Vishnu's advice. The great mountain, Mandara, was uprooted and used as a churning rod. Vasuki, the serpent king, served as a rope.

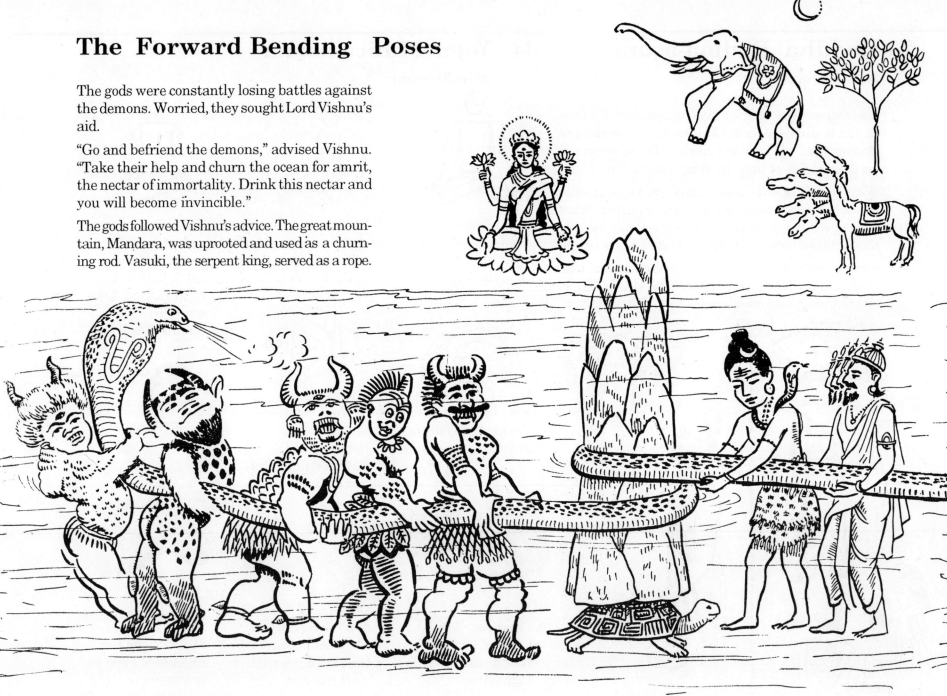

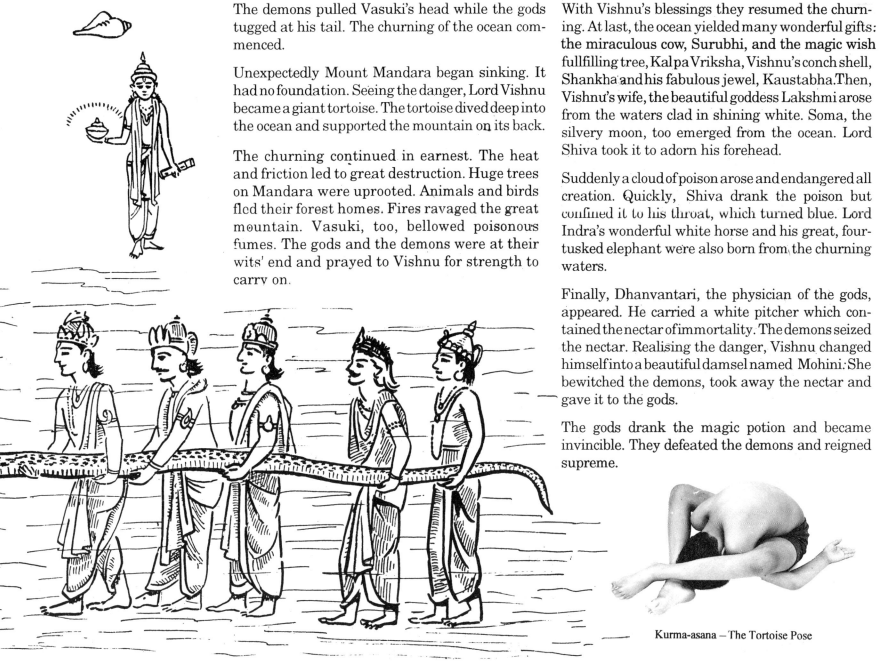

The demons pulled Vasuki's head while the gods tugged at his tail. The churning of the ocean commenced.

Unexpectedly Mount Mandara began sinking. It had no foundation. Seeing the danger, Lord Vishnu became a giant tortoise. The tortoise dived deep into the ocean and supported the mountain on its back.

The churning continued in earnest. The heat and friction led to great destruction. Huge trees on Mandara were uprooted. Animals and birds fled their forest homes. Fires ravaged the great mountain. Vasuki, too, bellowed poisonous fumes. The gods and the demons were at their wits' end and prayed to Vishnu for strength to carry on.

With Vishnu's blessings they resumed the churning. At last, the ocean yielded many wonderful gifts: the miraculous cow, Surubhi, and the magic wish fullfilling tree, Kalpa Vriksha, Vishnu's conch shell, Shankha and his fabulous jewel, Kaustabha. Then, Vishnu's wife, the beautiful goddess Lakshmi arose from the waters clad in shining white. Soma, the silvery moon, too emerged from the ocean. Lord Shiva took it to adorn his forehead.

Suddenly a cloud of poison arose and endangered all creation. Quickly, Shiva drank the poison but confined it to his throat, which turned blue. Lord Indra's wonderful white horse and his great, four-tusked elephant were also born from the churning waters.

Finally, Dhanvantari, the physician of the gods, appeared. He carried a white pitcher which contained the nectar of immortality. The demons seized the nectar. Realising the danger, Vishnu changed himself into a beautiful damsel named Mohini. She bewitched the demons, took away the nectar and gave it to the gods.

The gods drank the magic potion and became invincible. They defeated the demons and reigned supreme.

Kurma-asana – The Tortoise Pose

35. Danda-asana

20 to 40 counts

Danda means staff or rod. The spine is the axis of the human body. In Sanskrit it is called meru-danda.

Ancient texts describe a shining golden mountain named Meru, which is the axis of the universe. Brightly coloured birds, magical herbs, wishing-trees and precious stones abound on its slopes. This wonderful mountain is the home of many gods and heavenly beings.

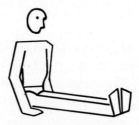

1. Sit on the floor. Extend your legs forward. Join your thighs, knees and big toes.

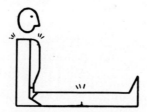

2. Place your palms on the floor beside your hips, fingers pointing forward. Expand your chest. Draw your shoulders back. This is *Danda-asana.*

DO

○ Keep your back as straight as a staff.

○ Tighten your knees, stretch the back of your legs.

○ Keep the soles of your feet well opened.

DON'T

☐ Don't lift your shoulders up.

BENEFITS

✿ Teaches you to sit correctly.

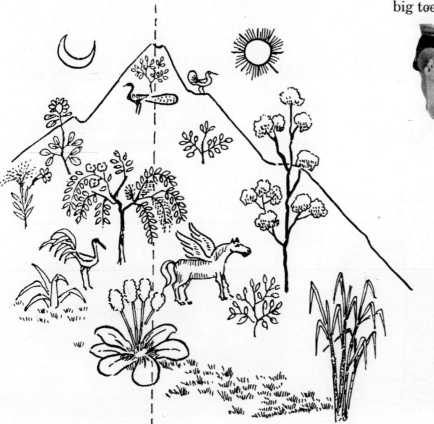

36. Janu Shirsha-asana

20 to 40 counts each side

Janu means knee and shirsha means head. In this pose you bring the head to the knee. In rural India women sit to grind grain in a pose similar to Janu Shirsha-asana. When they get tired they change their leg position and use the other arm. So by grinding grain they develop their body harmoniously. This action helps them to keep supple and healthy.

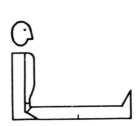

1. Sit in Danda-asana.

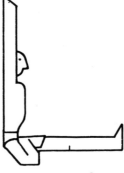

2. Bend your right knee and bring your right heel to your perineum. Raise your arms overhead.

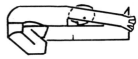

3. Bend forward. Hold your left foot with both hands. Lengthen your trunk. Rest your forehead or chin on your knees. This is Janu *Shirsha-asana.*

4. Then come up. Straighten your right leg and bend your left leg. Do the pose on the other side. Finally return to Danda-asana.

DO

○ Hold your ankle if you are stiff, gradually hold your foot.

○ Keep your extended leg poker stiff with your toes pointing upwards.

DON'T

☐ Don't keep one shoulder up and the other shoulder down, keep them level.

BENEFITS

✿ Stretches and strengthens the hamstring muscles.

✿ Tones the liver and kidneys.

✿ Rests the heart.

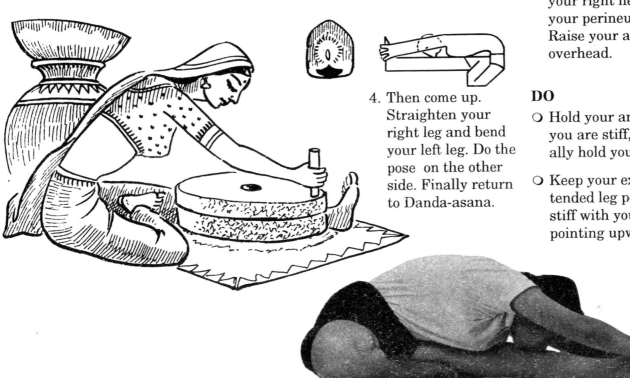

37. Ardha Baddha Padma Paschima-uttana-asana

20 to 40 counts each side

Ardha means half, baddha means restrained and Padma means lotus. Paschima-uttana-asana refers to the forward-bend in which the back body is stretched.

The lotus stands for purity and perfection. Many Indian gods and goddesses sit on a lotus seat. They often carry a lotus in one hand, and fold their legs in a half-lotus posture similar to Ardha Baddha Padma Paschima-uttana-asana.

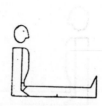

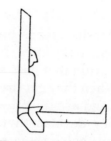

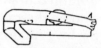

1. Sit in Danda-asana.

2. Bend your right knee as in Padma-asana. Keep your left leg straight with the toes pointing upwards. Raise your arms over-head.

3. Bend forward. Hold your left foot with both hands. Rest your forehead on your knee. This is *Ardha Baddha Padma Paschima-uttana-asana*.

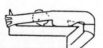

4. Then sit up. Straighten your right leg and bend your left knee. Repeat the pose on the other side. Finally return to Danda-asana.

DO
○ Lengthen the sides of your body.

DON'T
☐ Don't lift your knees off the floor.

BENEFITS
✿ Makes the knee joints strong and flexible.

✿ Makes the back supple.

✿ Strengthens the organs of the abdomen.

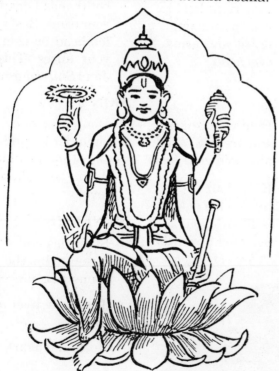

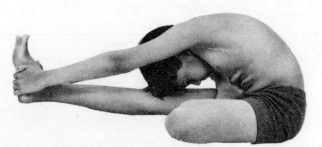

38. Tri-anga Mukha-ek-pada Paschima-uttana-asana

20 to 40 counts each side

Tri means three and anga means limbs. Mukha means face, ek means one and pada means leg. Paschima-uttana-asana refers to an intense stretch of the back. In this pose three limbs are kept extended while the face is brought to one leg.

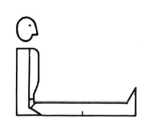

1. Sit in Danda-asana.

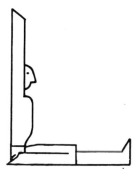

2. Bend your right knee back (as in Vira-asana). Keep your left leg poker stiff with the toes pointing upwards. Extend your arms overhead.

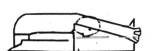

3. Lengthen your trunk. Bend forward. Hold your left foot. Rest your forehead on your knee. This is *Tri-anga Mukha-ek-pada Paschima-uttana-asana*.

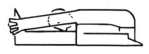

4. Then sit up. Straighten your right leg and bend your left leg back (as in Vira-asana). Repeat the pose. Finally return to Danda-asana.

DO

 Keep your shoulders parallel to the floor.

DON'T

 Don't tilt your body to a side.

BENEFITS

✿ Strengthens and shapes the legs.

✿ Makes the hip joints and the spine flexible.

✿ Exercises the muscles and organs of the abdomen.

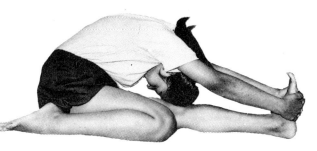

39. Marichi-asana I

20 to 40 counts each side

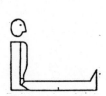

1. Sit in Danda-asana.

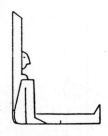

2. Bend your right knee upwards. Bring your right heel to your right buttock. Raise your arms overhead.

3. Then encircle your bent-knee with your right arm and take your left arm behind your back. Clasp hands.

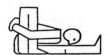

4. Bend forward. Rest your forehead on the extended knee. This is *Marichi-asana I*.

DO

○ Bring your armpit to the shin of your bent leg.

DON'T

□ Don't bring your knee towards your head, bring your head to your knee.

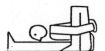

5. Then come up. Straighten out your right leg and bend your left knee upwards. Do the pose on the other side. Then return to Danda-asana.

BENEFITS

✿ Improves the digestion.

✿ Trims the waist.

Brahma, the creator, needed help in creating the universe. So by the power of his thought he created ten sages. Marichi was one of these great sages. These great sages made thirteen offerings to the fire-god. From these offerings men, horses, cows, sheep, barley, the rainy season and many other things were created.

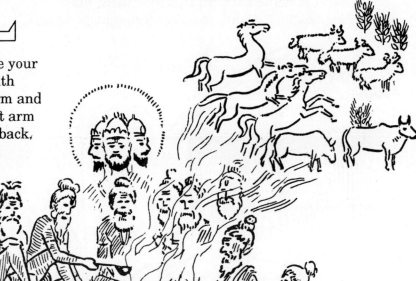

40. Marichi-asana II

20 to 40 counts each side

Sage Marichi was also the chief of the Marutas, the storm-gods. The storm-gods are the companions of Lord Indra. Armed with golden weapons, thunderbolts and lightning, they ride the winds and direct the storms.

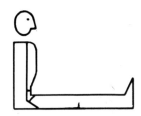

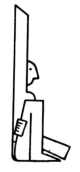

1. Sit in Danda-asana.

2. Bend your left leg as in Padma-asana. Then bend your right knee upwards. Raise your arms overhead.

3. Then encircle your right leg with your right arm and take your left arm behind your back. Clasp hands.

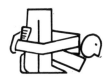

4. Bend forward. Rest your forehead or chin on your left knee. This is *Marichi-asana II*.

5. Then come up. Interchange the position of your legs. Do the pose on the other side. Finally return to Danda-asana.

DO

○ Bring your heel to your perineum when you bend your leg upwards.

DON'T

☐ Don't topple.

BENEFITS

✿ Makes the body flexible.

✿ Strengthens the lower abdomen.

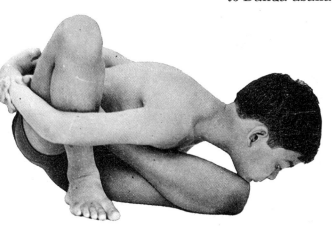

41. Paschima-uttana-asana

30 to 60 counts

Paschima means west and uttana means intense stretch. Indian sages have attributed directions to the human body. The top of the head is considered the north. The frontal body from the forehead to the toes is deemed the east. The soles of the feet are the south and the back of the body is considered the west.

In India the cardinal directions are of great importance. Priests, yogis and others always consider the compass points before commencing important activities. Ancient texts describe eight pairs of elephants who are the guardians of the eight directions.

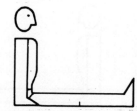

1. Sit in Danda-asana. Raise your arms over head. Lengthen your trunk.

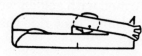

2. Bend forward. Hold your feet with both hands. Rest your forehead or chin on your knees. This is *Paschima-uttana-asana.*

DO

○ Stretch your back.

○ Join your big toes and broaden the soles of your feet.

DON'T

□ Don't bend your knees.

BENEFITS

✿ Invigorates the abdominal organs.

✿ Rests the heart.

✿ Refreshes the brain.

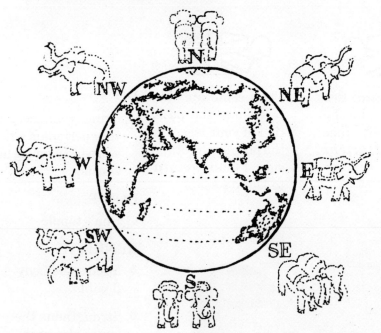

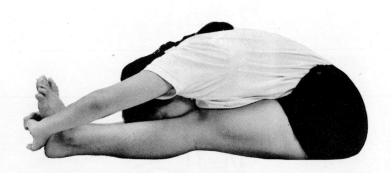

42. Baddha Kona-asana

30 to 60 counts each pose

Baddha means restrained and kona means an angle. Indian cobblers sit in this position while mending shoes. In the fifteenth century A.D. there lived a wise cobbler in North India. He was called Sant Ravidas. Renowned as he was for his wisdom, he continued to work as a cobbler. One day a great king came to seek his blessings. Promptly. Ravidas offered the king some water from the bowl in which he soaked leather. The king was revolted. He pretended to drink the water but spilt it down the front of his shirt.

The washerwoman at the palace learned of the king's deceit. She took the king's wet shirt, wrung out a few drops of water, and drank them. Having thus received Ravidas's blessings, she became a wise woman.

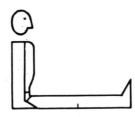

1. Sit in Danda-asana.

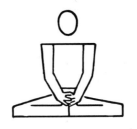

2. Bend your knees sideways. Join the soles of your feet. Broaden your chest and draw your shoulders back. Sit erect. This is *Baddha Kona-asana*.

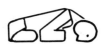

3. Then bend forward. Rest your forehead or chin on the floor. This is *Baddha Kona-asana II*.

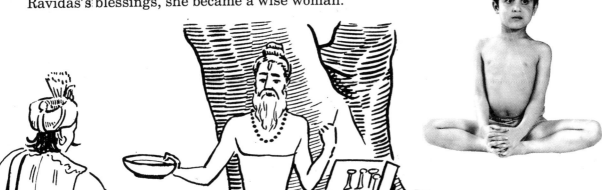

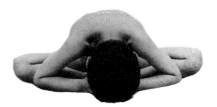

DO
○ Pull your heels in towards your perineum.

DON'T
☐ Don't raise your knees off the floor.

BENEFITS
✿ Keeps the hip and knee joints healthy.
✿ Improves the functioning of lower abdominal organs.
✿ Increases control over the bladder.

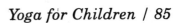

43. Upavista Kona-asana

20 to 40 counts each pose

Upavista means seated and kona means angle. Modern lifestyle confines and limits our movements. We sit in a similar position all day at the dining table, in cars, in buses, at school, at the movies, watching TV... While practising Yoga-asanas like Upavista Kona-asana we explore a wide range of movements. This keeps our joints, muscles, organs and nerves strong and healthy.

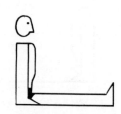

1. Sit in Danda-asana.

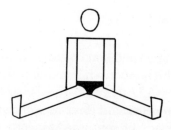

2. Widen your legs sideways, one leg at a time. Tighten the muscles of your legs and keep your toes pointing upwards. Sit erect.

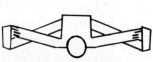

3. Hook your big toes with your index and middle fingers. Bend forward. Rest your forehead or chin on the floor. This is *Upavista Kona-asana*.

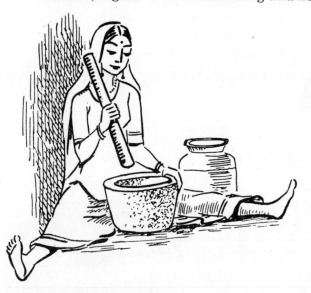

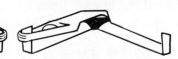

4. Then rotate your waist to your left. Hold your left foot with both hands. Rest your chin or forehead on your left knee. Sit up as in number 2.

5. Rotate your waist to your right. Hold your right foot with both hands. Rest your forehead or chin on your right knee. This is *Upavista Kona-asana II*. Finally return to Danda-asana.

DO

○ Spread your legs as wide as you can.

DON'T

☐ Don't bend your knees.

BENEFITS

✿ Improves circulation in the pelvic region.

✿ Makes the hamstring muscles elastic.

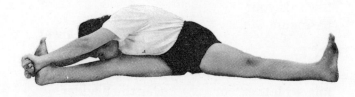

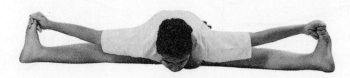

44. Kurma-asana

20 to 40 counts

45. Supta Kurma-asana

20 to 40 counts

Kurma means tortoise. Seeing that Mount Mandara had no foundation and was sinking, Lord Vishnu became a giant tortoise. The tortoise dived into the ocean and lifted the mountain up on its back. The tortoise was very strong and raised the mountain too high. To set things right, Vishnu also became an eagle. The eagle sat on top of Mount Mandara and pushed it into place. Then the churning of the ocean continued. Supta means sleeping. In Supta Kurma-asana you withdraw your limbs like a sleeping tortoise.

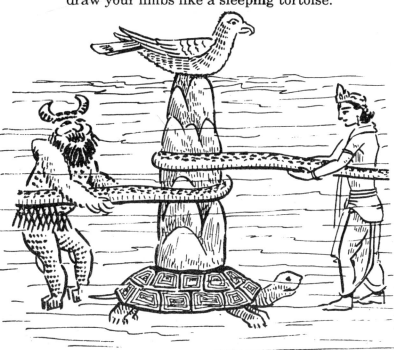

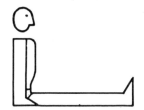

1. Sit in Danda-asana.

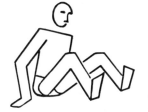

2. Bend your knees upwards. Spread your feet about eighteen inches.

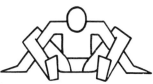

3. Insert your arms under your knees. Extend your arms sideways.

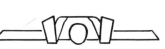

4. Now try to straighten your legs without widening them too much. Rest your head, chin or chest on the floor. This is *Kurma-asana.*

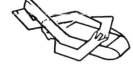

5. Bend your elbows. Clasp hands behind your back. Then cross your ankles. Rest your head on the floor between your legs. This is *Supta Kurma-asana.*

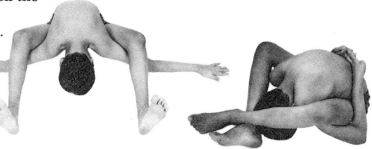

DO

O Place your knees over your shoulders.

DON'T

☐ Don't forget to interchange the position of your crossed ankles and clasped hands.

BENEFITS

✿ Makes the spine supple.

✿ Soothes and quietens the mind.

The Twisting Poses

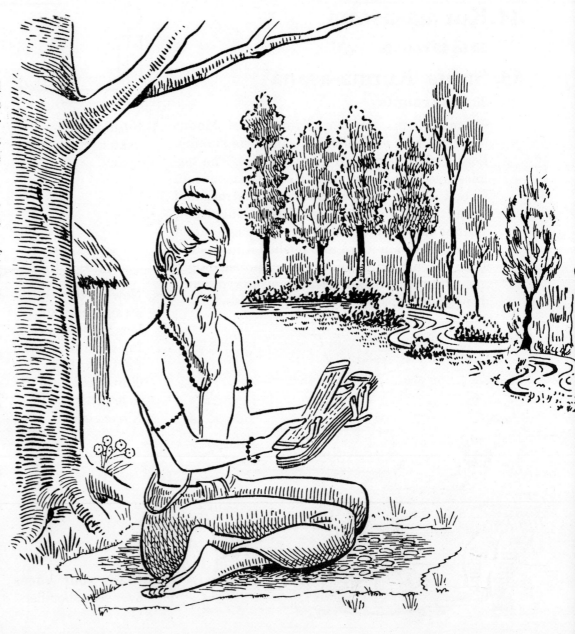

When the Earth was young there lived a good and wise sage named Bharadvaja. He spent most of his days studying the Vedic scriptures. His thirst for learning knew no bounds. He soon realised that the great scriptures could not be mastered in one lifetime.

Bharadvaja decided to invoke Lord Indra's blessings for a long life. In a quiet place in the forest he practised severe penance for many years. "Grant me, O Lord," he pleaded, " a lifetime of many thousands of years so that I may study the Vedas." Pleased, Lord Indra granted him his wish.

With one pointed attention Bharadvaja continued his study of the Vedas. Thousands of years went by but his studies remained incomplete. Realising that this long life was coming to an end Bharadvaja again prayed to Indra. "O Lord," he beseeched, "I need several thousand years more to complete my task."

Lord Indra appeared before his devotee. He took him before three mountains. Then picking up three handfuls of sand Indra gave them to Bharadvaja. "What you have learned so far only amounts to these three handfuls of sand," said Indra. "The Vedas yet to be studied are equal to these three mountains."

Bharadvaja was not to be discouraged. He accepted the challenge and continued his studies undaunted.

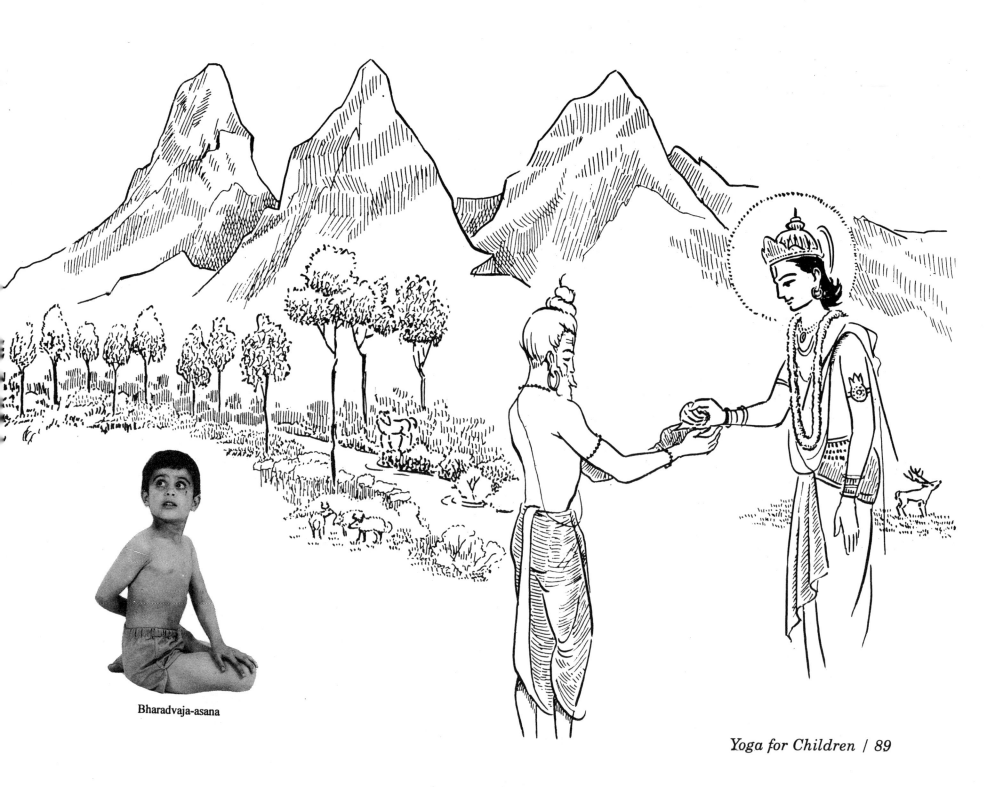

Bharadvaja-asana

46. Bharadvaja-asana I

20 to 30 counts each side

Bharadvaja was a great rishi. Sages and men of great wisdom were called rishis. Rishis lived in hermitages or ashrams along with their family and devoted students. Ashrams were usually located in deep forests on quiet mountains.

Rishis differed in nature. Some were poets and philosophers. Some were healers. Some were ascetics. Some were prone to fits of anger, even the gods feared the curse of a rishi. Often rishis had magical powers.

Rishi Bharadvaja had his ashram at Prayag where the holy rivers Ganga and Yamuna meet. There he and his pupils led a disciplined life devoted to study and religious practices.

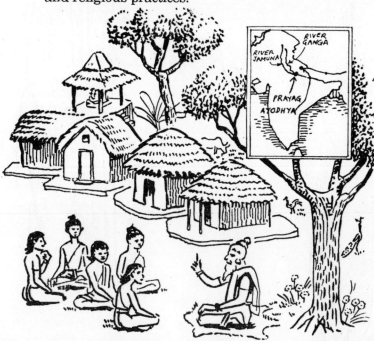

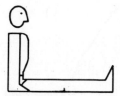

1. Sit in Danda-asana.

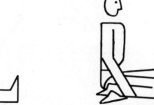

2. Bend your legs back. Place both feet beside your right hip. Keep your right ankle over the arch of the left foot.

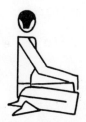

3. Hold your left knee with your right hand.

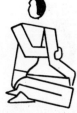

4. Swing your left arm behind your back. Catch hold of your right arm. Turn your head. Look over your left shoulder. This is *Bharadvaja-asana I*.

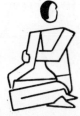

5. Then straighten your legs. Interchange the position of your legs, feet and arms. Do the pose on the other side. Finally return to Danda-asana.

DO
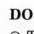
- Turn your head, shoulders, waist and elbows.

DON'T
- Don't move your knees while turning.

BENEFITS
- Relieves sore backs and stiff necks.

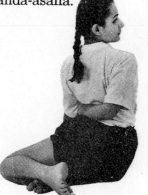
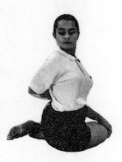

47. Bharadvaja-asana II

20 to 30 seconds each side

During their exile Rama, Sita and Lakshmana sought shelter at Rishi Bharadvaja's ashram in Prayag. Bharadvaja greeted them warmly and showered them with hospitality. Before their departure he advised them where they could spend their days in the forest.

Fourteen years later Lord Rama and his companions were returning from exile to their home in Ayodhya. They had defeated Ravana, the wicked king of Lanka. To greet the victorious Rama, Bharadvaja cast a magic spell. He made every tree between Prayag and Ayodhya burst into blossom! Such was the power of Bharadvaja's magic.

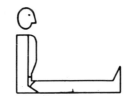

1. Sit in Danda-asana.

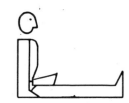

2. Bend your left leg as in Padma-asana.

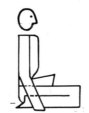

3. Bend your right leg as in Vira-asana.

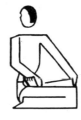

4. Swing your left arm behind your back and catch hold of your left foot.

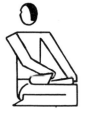

5. Then hold your left knee with your right hand. Turn your head. Look over your left shoulder. This is *Bharadvaja asana II*.

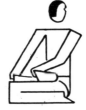

6. Then straighten out your legs. Interchange the position of your legs and arms and do the pose on the other side. Finally return to Danda-asana.

DO

○ Turn your shoulders and look as far back as you can.

DON'T

☐ Don't despair if you can't reach your foot, hold your T-shirt instead.

BENEFITS

✿ Improves stiff shoulders and knees.

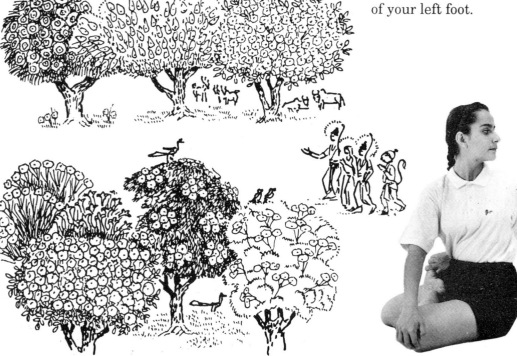

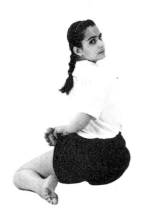

48. Marichi-asana III

20 to 30 counts each side

Marichi was a sage. He was the son of Brahma, the creator. His name means ray-of-light. Sage Marichi is identified with one of the bright stars in the constellation Ursa Major (the Great Bear).

The seven bright stars of Ursa Major are called Sapta Rishi or Seven Sages in India. Six of these shining sages are married to the six Pleiadies. The seventh sage is married to Arundhiti, the morning star.

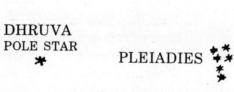

DHRUVA
POLE STAR

PLEIADIES

SEVEN SAGES
URSA MAJOR.

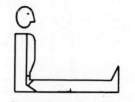

1. Sit in Danda-asana.

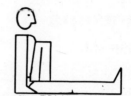

2. Bend your left knee upwards. Keep your right leg poker stiff.

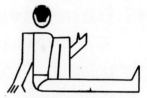

3. Rotate your waist to your left. Fix your right shoulder outside your left knee. Keep your left fingertips on the floor.

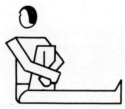

4. Then curl your right arm around your left shin. Swing your left arm behind your back and clasp the right hand.

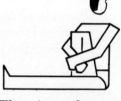

5. Turn your head and look over your left shoulder. Twist your waist and move your left shoulder further back. This is *Marichi-asana III*.

6. Then interchange the position of your legs and arms. Now do the pose turning to your right. Finally return to Danda-asana.

DO
○ Bring your armpit to your knee while entwining.

DON'T
☐ Don't despair if you can't clasp hands, hold your T-shirt instead.

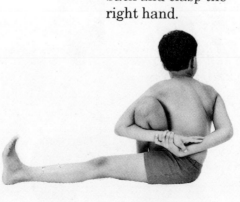

BENEFITS
✿ Trims the waist.

✿ Relieves backaches and stiff necks.

✿ Improves appetite.

49. Pasha-asana

20 to 30 counts each side

Pasha means noose or cord. In this pose you make a noose of your arms and tie yourself. Pasha is the dreaded weapon used by Pashin, the God of Righteousness. Pashin catches and binds wicked people with his noose. No one can escape from him because he knows what is in the hearts of men.

Pashin is also known as Varuna, the lord of the ocean. He rides on a sea monster called Makara. (See Makara-asana).

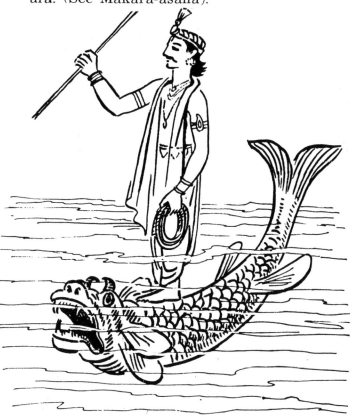

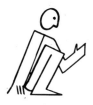

1. Squat. Use a folded blanket under the heels if your can't balance. Join your feet.

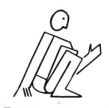

2. Rotate your waist to your left. Fix your right upper arm on the outer side of your left knee. Keep your left fingertips on the floor.

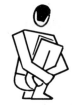

3. Then curl your right arm around your shins. Swing your left arm behind your back and clasp your right hand.

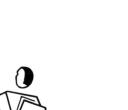

4. Turn your head, look over your left shoulder. Twist your waist and move your left elbow and shoulder further back. This is *Pasha-asana*.

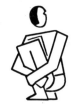

5. Loosen your arms. Now do the pose turning to your right side.

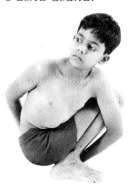

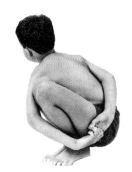

DO
○ Tighten the noose.

DON'T
☐ Don't clasp hands under your buttocks, clasp behind your back.

BENEFITS
✿ Corrects round shoulders.
✿ Strengthens spinal muscles, soothes sore backs.
✿ Improves appetite, digestion and elimination.

50. Ardha Matsyendra-asana I

20 to 30 counts each side

Matsyendra was a great yogi. His name means Fish-Lord. Once Lord Shiva and his wife Parvati were sitting by the sea. Shiva was explaining the mysterious philosophy of Yoga to his wife. Finding the explanations too difficult, Parvati fell asleep. A clever little fish had keenly heard every word spoken by Shiva. Noticing this, Shiva made the little fish into a great yogi named Matsyendranath.

Ardha means half. This pose is a simple variation of a more difficult pose called Paripoorna (full) Matsyendra-asana.

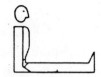

1. Sit in Danda-asana.

2. Bend your right leg in. Sit on your right foot.

3. Bend your left knee upwards. Take your left foot across your right knee.

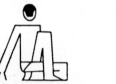

4. Rotate your waist to your left. Fix your right upper arm against your left outer knee. Rest your left fingertips on the floor.

5. Curl your right arm around your left shin. Then swing your left arm behind your back and clasp your right hand.

6. Turn your head and look over your left shoulder. This is *Ardha Matsyendra-asana I*.

Then interchange the position of your arms and legs. Do the pose on the other side. Finally return to Danda-asana.

DO
○ Lift up your stomach as you turn.

DON'T
☐ Don't leave a gap between your bent-knee and your armpit.

BENEFITS
✿ Prevents and cures backaches.

✿ Tones the liver, spleen and pancreas.

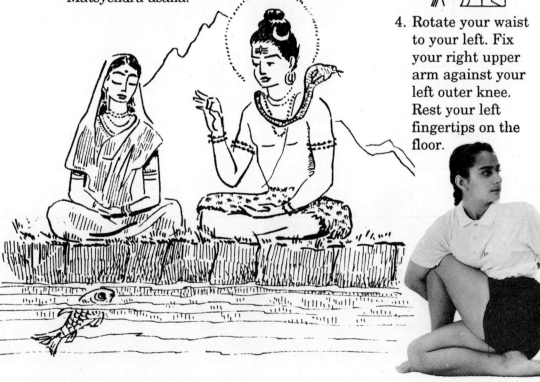

51. Ardha Matsyendra-asana II

20 to 30 counts each side

Sage Matsyendra lived at the end of the tenth century A.D. He was famed for his magical powers. He and his followers were called Natha Yogis. Natha Yogis were powerful magicians. Folk tales tell that they could command the rain to fall. They could assume different forms. They could fly in the air and could control wild animals. Natha Yogis, it is said, could live for hundreds of years. Some people say that Natha Yogis still live in remote Himalayan caves.

Ardha means half. This pose prepares you for Paripoorna (full) Matsyendra-asana.

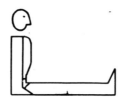

1. Sit in Danda-asana.

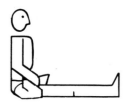

2. Bend your right leg as in Padma-asana.

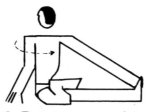

3. Rotate your waist to your left. Hold your left foot with your right hand.

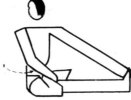

4. Throw your left arm behind your back and catch hold of your right ankle. Look over your left shoulder. This is *Ardha Matsyendra-asana II.*

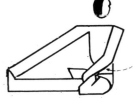

5. Then interchange the position of your legs and arms. Now do the pose turning to your right side. Finally return to Danda-asana.

DO

○ Twist your stomach.

DON'T

☐ Don't hold your breath.

BENEFITS

✿ Makes the spine strong and supple.

✿ Corrects drooping shoulders.

✿ Tones the abdominal organs.

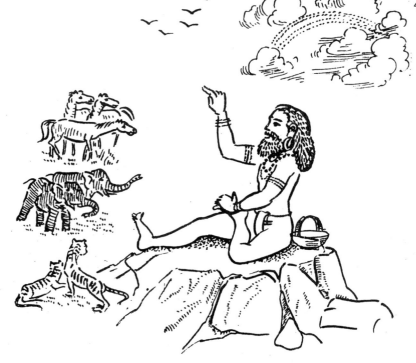

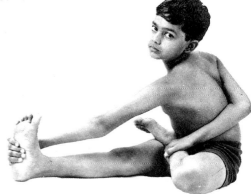

The Backward Bending Poses

One day the young Kaurava and Pandava princes were playing with a ball. Their ball rolled away and fell into a well. The boys gathered around the well wondering what to do. Then they noticed a lean and dark brahmin sitting under a tree. They sought his help.

"Will you reward me if I retrieve your ball?" asked the brahmin.

"Yes, yes, certainly!" said the boys, eager to resume their game.

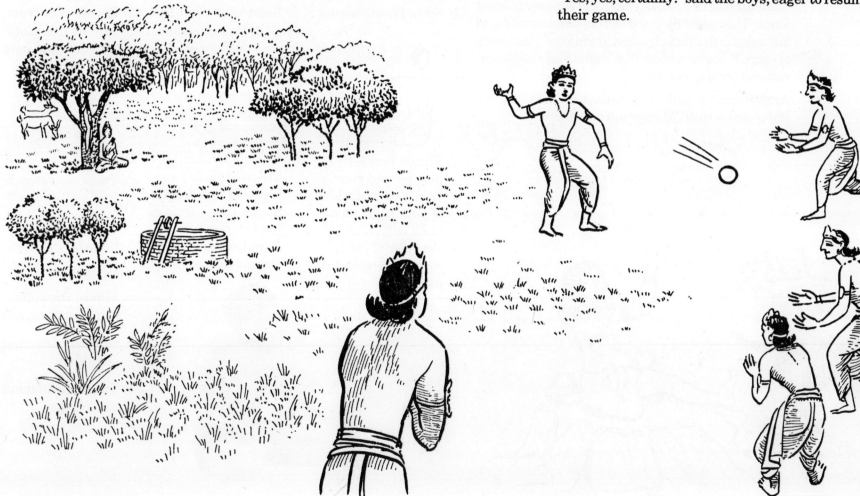

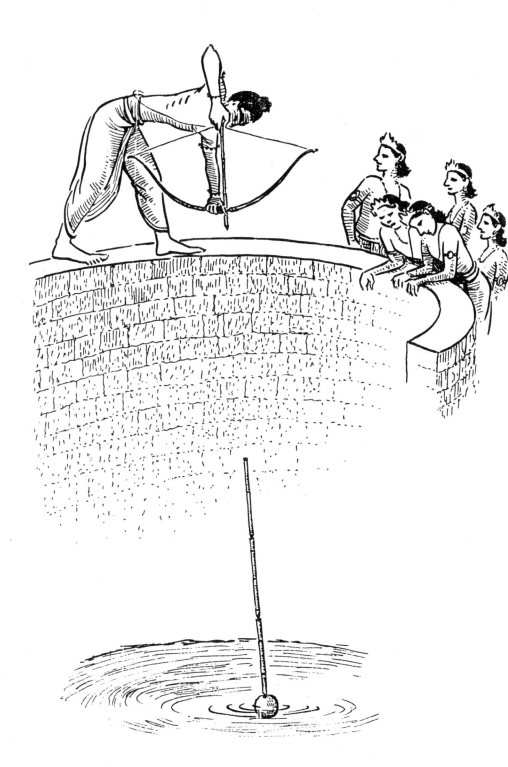

The brahmin asked for a bow. He then plucked some sharp reeds growing near the well. Using a reed as an arrow, he shot it straight at the ball. He shot another reed behind it and then several more, till they formed a chain. With this chain he drew the ball out of the well.

The astonished princes bowed before the archer. "How can we reward such a great feat?" they asked each other.

Seeing this the brahmin said, "Go to your grand-uncle, Bhishma, and tell him what happened."

The boys went running to Bhishma and described the archer's feat. The wise Bhishma realised that this great archer could be none other than Drona, the son of Sage Bharadvaja. He immediately called Drona and appointed him to teach the young princes archery and warfare.

Under Drona's able guidance the princes grew up to be renowned warriors.

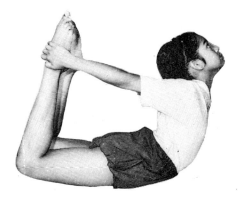

Dhanur-asana-The Bow Pose

52. Shalabha-asana

10 to 15 counts

Shalabha means grasshopper or locust. The sages of ancient India lived close to nature. They carefully observed the natural world around them and studied the behaviour of various creatures. They realised that man could learn many secrets of health and rejuvenation from nature. No wonder numerous asanas are derived from nature: mountains, trees, animals, reptiles, birds and even an insect, the grasshopper!

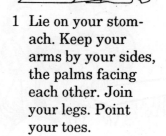

1 Lie on your stomach. Keep your arms by your sides, the palms facing each other. Join your legs. Point your toes.

2 Raise your head, chest, legs and arms off the floor simultaneously. *This is Shalabha-asana*

DO

○ Imagine you are a grasshopper, your arms are your wings.

DON'T

☐ Don't let your thighs touch the floor.

☐ Don't bend your knees.

BENEFITS

✿ Strengthens the muscles of the back, the hips and the back of the thighs.

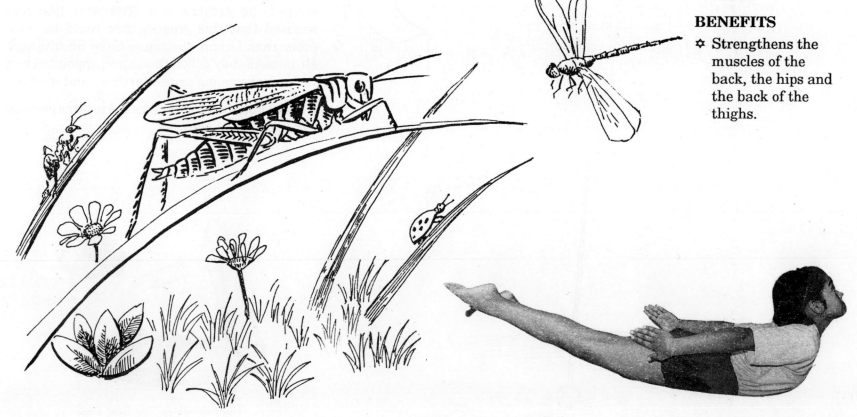

53. Makara-asana

10 to 15 counts

Makara is a mythological sea-creature. It has the head and forelegs of a horned beast, and the body and tail of a fish. Varuna, the Lord of the Ocean, rides on Makara. The zodiac constellation Capricorn is also called Makara.

1 Lie on your stomach. Interlock your fingers behind your head. Join your legs. Point your toes.

2 Raise your head, chest and legs off the floor simultaneously. *This is Makara-asana.*

DO

○ Imagine you are Makara, your elbows are your horns.

DON'T

☐ Don't let your thighs remain on the floor.

☐ Don't bend your knees.

BENEFITS

✿ Strengthens the muscles of the back, the neck and back of the thighs.

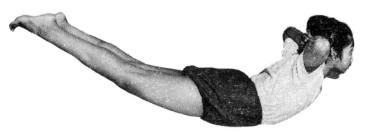

54. Bhujanga-asana

10 to 15 counts

Bhujanga means a snake. The mightiest among snakes is the snake king, Vasuki. To churn the ocean the gods needed Vasuki to serve as a rope. They requested the mighty eagle, Garuda, to bring Vasuki to the seashore. Eager to display his strength, the proud Garuda set off.

On finding the great snake, Garuda said, "O Vasuki, the gods require your service urgently!"

"I will be happy to help the gods," replied Vasuki, "but you will have to carry me to the seashore."

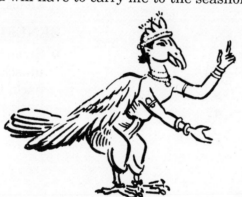

Garuda promptly grabbed the snake's middle in his huge claws and flew off. He ascended higher and higher till he reached the heavens. Looking down, Garuda was astonished. Vasuki's head and coiled tail were still on the ground far below! Humbled, Garuda returned to the gods.

Then Lord Shiva lowered his arm. Vasuki coiled himself into a bracelet on Shiva's wrist. Lord Shiva then took Vasuki to the seashore.

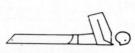

1 Lie on your stomach. Join your legs. Point your toes. Place your palms to the sides of your chest with the fingers well spread and pointing forward.

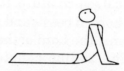

2 Raise your trunk off the floor. Straighten your arms. Throw your head back. Arch your spine as much as possible. This is *Bhujanga-asana*.

DO

○ Puff out your chest, take your head back like a cobra about to strike.

○ Tighten the muscles of your thighs.

DON'T

☐ Don't raise your thighs off the floor.

BENEFITS

✡ Helps remove stiffness in the neck and spine.

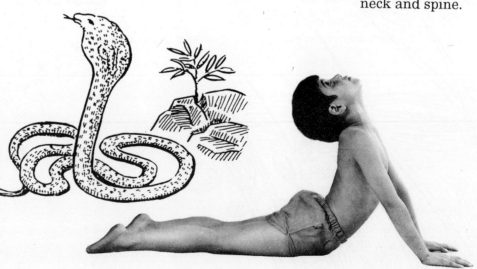

55. Ushtra-asana

10 to 15 counts

Ushtra means camel. A camel and a jackal were once good friends. One night they sneaked into a sugar cane field. Having eaten his fill, the jackal began howling.

"Stop! Stop!" whispered the camel. "Your howling will wake up the farmer."

The selfish jackal continued howling. When the farmer arrived, the sly jackal hid in the bushes. The camel got a good beating.

Fleeing, the friends came to a river. The jackal climbed up on the camel's back. In the middle of the river the camel said, "I want to take a dip."

"Don't do that, pleaded the jackal. "I can't swim! I shall drown."

The camel promptly took a dip. The jackal nearly drowned. The kind camel rescued him and brought him ashore. So the camel taught the selfish jackal a lesson.

Remember, the wise sages taught *selflessness*, not *selfishness*.

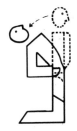

1 Kneel with your toes pointing backwards. Rest your hands on your hips. Curve back.

2 Drop your palms one by one, onto the soles of your feet. This is *Ushtra-asana*. Then come up, bringing one hand up at a time.

DO
- Push your tailbone forward.
- Stretch your neck.

DON'T
- Don't look up, instead look down.

BENEFITS
- Helps remove stiffness in the neck and shoulders.

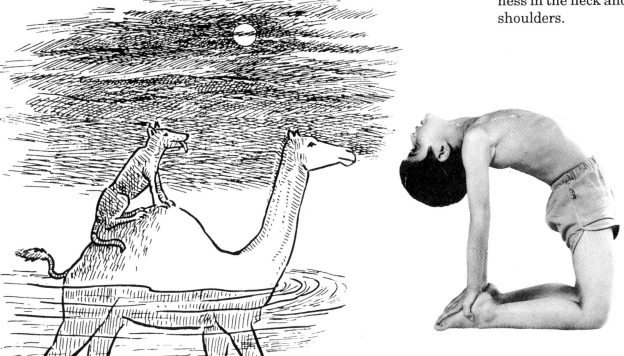

56. Dhanur-asana

10 to 15 counts

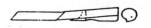

1. Lie on your stomach.

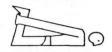

2. Bend your knees. Hold your ankles.

3. Raise your thighs, head and chest off the floor. This is *Dhanur-asana*.

DO

○ Bring your head closer to your feet.

○ Curve your body like a bow, stretch your arms like the bow string.

DON'T

□ Don't let your ribs or your thighs remain on the floor.

Dhanu means bow. In ancient India there once lived a beautiful princess named Draupadi. To find her a suitable husband, her father, King Drupada, decided to hold an archery contest. Many great princes and warriors flocked to the King's court hoping to win fair Draupadi's hand. Amongst these were Drona's pupils, the brave Pandava princes. As these princes were in exile, they came in disguise.

On the day of the contest all the suitors assembled in a great hall at the palace. King Drupada had set a formidable challenge before them. A large and heavy bow had been made especially for the occasion. The target was a revolving metal fish set atop a high pole. The pole was placed in a pool of water. The archers were not to look directly at the target, but at the reflection of the target in the pool below. Whosoever shot five arrows through the eye of this revolving fish would win fair Draupadi for his bride.

The contest began. One by one several famed heroes strode up to the bow, only to return disappointed. Despite their prowess, this task proved too difficult for them.

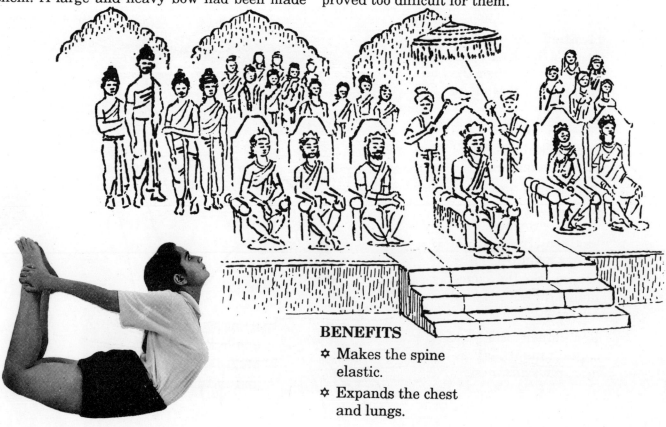

BENEFITS

✿ Makes the spine elastic.

✿ Expands the chest and lungs.

57. Urdhva Dhanur-asana

10 to 15 counts

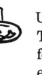

Urdhva means upwards or raised and dhanur means bow. Then a tall, handsome stranger walked up to the bow. With folded palms he prayed to Lord Vishnu to assist him in his endeavour. He then easily lifted the mighty bow and rapidly shot five arrows through the eye of the revolving fish.

Delighted, Draupadi garlanded the victor accepting him as her husband!

This stranger was, in fact, the Pandava prince, Arjuna, the greatest archer in the land.

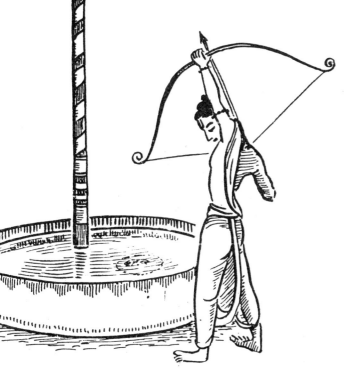

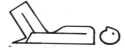

1 Lie on your back. Bend your knees. Bring your heels to your hips. Keep your feet about eight inches apart and parallel to each other.

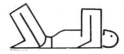

2 Place your palms under your shoulders. The fingers must point towards your feet.

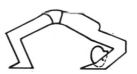

3 Raise your back and buttocks off the floor. Curve your spine and rest the crown of your head on the floor.

4 Now straighten your arms. Then walk towards your hands and arch your spine further. This is *Urdhva Dhanur-asana.* Then bend your elbows and come down gently.

DO

○ Bend your body like a bow.

DON'T

☐ Don't bend your elbows.

☐ Don't widen your knees too much.

BENEFITS

✿ Corrects rounded back and shoulders.

✿ Improves respiration.

✿ Removes dullness and laziness.

✿ Makes you strong and energetic.

58 Kapota-asana

10 to 15 counts

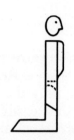
1. Kneel with your toes pointing backwards.

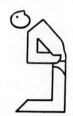
2. Rest your hands on your hips. Curve back.

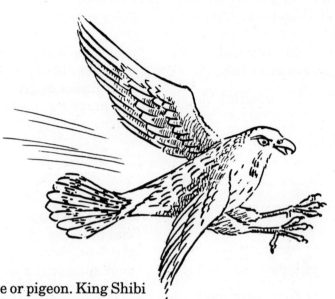

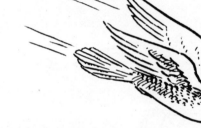

Kapota means a dove or pigeon. King Shibi was a good and just ruler. He cared for all of his subjects and was kind to animals, too. His fame spread on earth and in heaven.

One day, a dove, which was fleeing from a hawk, took shelter on King Shibi's lap. "Don't worry, little dove," assured the gentle king, "you are safe with me."

Angrily, the hawk swooped down. "Give me the dove," it demanded. "I am hungry! By protecting the dove you are being unjust to me."

I shall give you the meat of a deer or a boar instead," said King Shibi.

"I don't eat deer or boar," replied the hawk. "The dove is my natural prey."

"Please spare this dove," begged the King. "You can ask for anything else you wish."

"Flesh from your body equal to the weight of the dove is the only other food which I shall accept!"

King Shibi did not hesitate. He sent for a pair of scales and a knife. He placed the dove on one pan of the scale and on the other pan he placed chunks of his own flesh. Though he carved out many pieces of flesh from his legs and arms, still the dove remained heavier. Then, seeing no other option, King Shibi stepped onto the scales.

"Eat me," said the King to the hawk.

Instantly, the hawk turned into Lord Indra and the dove changed into Lord Agni, the God of Fire.

King Shibi had passed the severe test put to him by the gods. Pleased with Shibi's sacrifice, the gods blessed him and made him whole again.

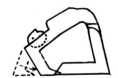

3. Curve further. Take your arms over your head. Drop your palms on the floor or onto your feet.

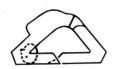

4. Grip your toes or your heels with your hands. Rest your head and elbows on the floor. This is *Kapota-asana*.

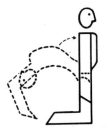

5. Then return to the kneeling position with a swing.

DO

○ Puff out your chest like a dove.

DON'T

☐ Don't widen your knees too much.

BENEFITS

✿ Makes the spine strong and flexible.

✿ Strengthens the heart and lungs.

✿ Makes you courageous.

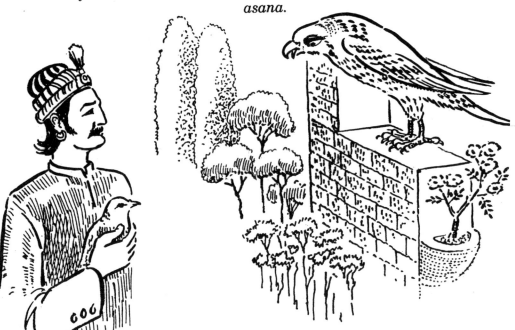

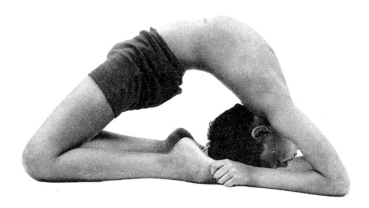

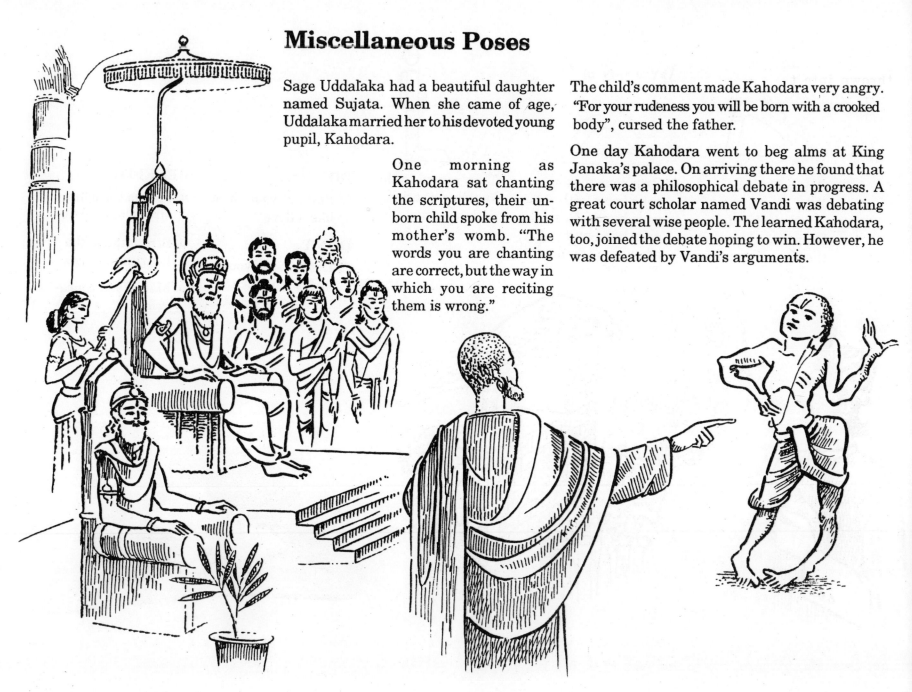

Miscellaneous Poses

Sage Uddaḷaka had a beautiful daughter named Sujata. When she came of age, Uddalaka married her to his devoted young pupil, Kahodara.

One morning as Kahodara sat chanting the scriptures, their unborn child spoke from his mother's womb. "The words you are chanting are correct, but the way in which you are reciting them is wrong."

The child's comment made Kahodara very angry. "For your rudeness you will be born with a crooked body", cursed the father.

One day Kahodara went to beg alms at King Janaka's palace. On arriving there he found that there was a philosophical debate in progress. A great court scholar named Vandi was debating with several wise people. The learned Kahodara, too, joined the debate hoping to win. However, he was defeated by Vandi's arguments.

The proud victor demanded that Kahodara be thrown into the river. Kahodara drowned and died.

Shortly thereafter, the widowed Sujata gave birth to a boy. The boy was born with eight bends in his body. So he was named Ashtavakra, he-who-has eight-bends.

Though bent and crooked, Ashtavakra grew up to be a bright and clever young boy. When he was twelve, he came to know how his father died.

The spirited boy vowed to avenge his father's death and set off for Janaka's palace. Although he was a child, Ashtavakra challenged and defeated the learned Vandi in a debate. He then demanded that the haughty scholar be thrown into the river.

When Janaka's soldiers threw Vandi into the river, a miracle occured. Ashtavakra's father, Kahodara, arose from the river and came back to life!

Delighted, Kahodara hugged and blessed his son. Then he took Ashtavakra to bathe in a river. After a bath Ashtavakra discovered that he was not crooked anymore. His limbs were straight and beautiful!

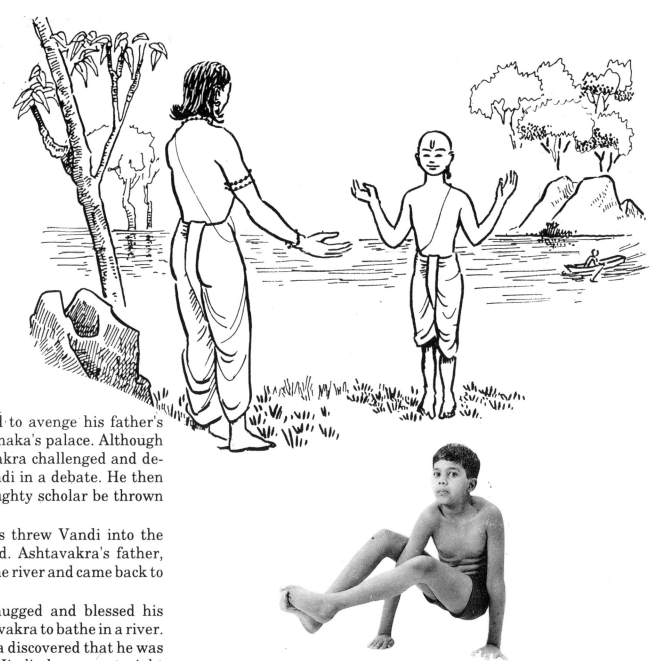

Ashta-vakra-asana

59. Vira-asana I 1 to 2 minutes
60. Vira-asana II 30 to 60 counts

Vira means a warrior or a hero. The great epic Mahabharata tells of many great warriors and heroes. Perhaps the greatest amongst them was Bhishma, the patriarch and teacher of the Kaurava and Pandava clans.

When war between the cousins became inevitable, the dutiful Bhishma remained with the Kauravas. He was appointed the commander of their army. For nine days Bhishma led his forces with great skill and valour. The Pandava army could not match his strategy and courage.

The Pandavas were desperate. That evening they sent their leader Yudhisthira to meet Bhishma. "O mighty Guru," Yudhisthira implored, "help us, our cause is just!"

Well aware that the Pandavas were fighting for a righteous cause, Bhishma said, "You must first kill me if you wish to win this battle. There is only one way of doing this.

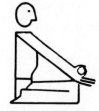

1. Sit on the floor with both legs bent back. Your hips must rest on the floor between your feet. Join your knees.

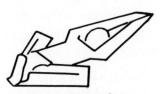

2. Perform the Jnana Mudra by joining the tips of the index fingers with the tips of the thumbs. Sit erect. Look straight. This is *Vira-asana*.

3. Then spread your knees wide apart and join your big toes. Bend forward. Rest your forehead on the floor and stretch out your arms. This is *Vira-asana II*

I shall not fight a woman, so send a woman warrior to fight against me!".
The next day the Pandavas deployed a female warrior named Shikhandi against Bhishma. Arjuna followed close behind Shikhandi in his chariot. Bhishma refused to take up arms against the woman. Arjuna seized this opportunity. Rapidly, he shot many arrows at Bhishma. Thus the mighty warrior, Bhishma, fell.

DO
O Draw your shoulders back and sit straight like a warrior.

DON'T
❑ Don't turn your feet sideways.

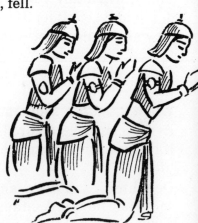

BENEFITS
☆ Corrects flat feet and strengthens the ankles.
☆ Removes pain, cramps and fatigue in the legs, good for sportsmen.
☆ Makes the knee joint flexible and strong.
☆ Aids digestion.

61. Supta Vira-asana

2 to 4 minutes

Supta means sleeping and vira means a warrior or hero.

When Bhishma fell under Arjuna's shower of arrows, his body did not hit the ground. It remained aloft on a bed of arrows! Still, the mighty Bhishma did not die. He even refused to be removed from the battlefield and to have his wounds tended. "A bed of arrows befits a dying warrior," he remarked.

The furious battle raged on. However, around Bhishma's bed there was calm. The Kaurava and the Pandava princes, great kings and noblemen came to his side. They begged his forgiveness and sought his advice on state-craft and right conduct. For fifty-nine days Bhishma lay thus.

Then, at an auspicious moment, the brave, old warrior who had the power to decide the time of his death, chose to breathe his last. His spirit departed to heaven.

1. Sit in Vira-asana.

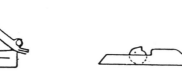

2. Supporting yourself with your elbows, lie back. Extend your arms overhead. This is *Supta Vira-asana*.

DO

○ Keep your toes pointing back as i the photo.

○ Lengthen your trunk.

DON'T

☐ Don't lie back on your heels.

☐ Don't widen your knees.

☐ Don't arch your back.

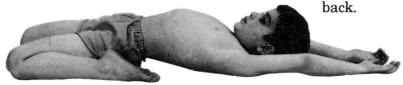

BENEFITS

✿ Removes fatigue and refreshes the body.

✿ Helps to breathe deeply.

✿ Rests the heart.

✿ Helps relieve stomach problems.

✿ Calms and quietens the mind.

62. Go-mukha-asana

10 to 15 counts each side

Go means cow and mukha means mouth or face. In this asana the gap between the knees resembles a cow's mouth.

In an agrarian society like India, the cow is a very useful animal. Cows provide milk for food. Bulls are a very useful source of animal power. They plough the fields and transport goods. Cowdung is a good natural fertilizer. Even dead the cow is useful by providing leather.

No wonder Indian legends describe a wish-fulfilling cow called Kamadhenu. It was born from the churning of the ocean. One could milk it for whatever one wanted.

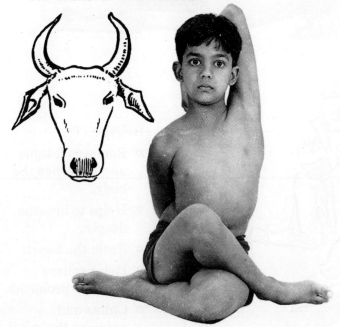

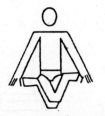

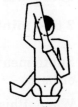

1. Sit on the floor. Fold your left leg in. Then fold your right leg over the left so that one knee is above the other.

2. Take your left arm over your head and bend it at the elbow. Place the left hand between your shoulder-blades.

3. Then take your right hand behind your back. Hook the fingers of your left hand with the fingers of the right hand. This is *Go-mukha-asana*.

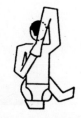

4. Interchange the position of your legs and arms and repeat the pose.

DO

○ Look straight ahead.

○ Keep one elbow pointing to the ceiling and the other elbow pointing to the ground.

DON'T

☐ Don't stoop forward.

BENEFITS

✿ Relieves cramps in the calves.

✿ Improves stiff and rounded shoulders.

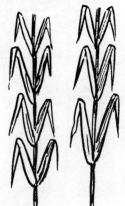

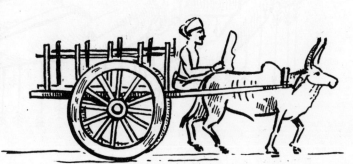

63. Lola-asana

5 to 10 counts

Lola means dangling or moving back and forth, like a swing. Indians are very fond of swings. Ancient tales describe how gods and goddesses sit on swings in heavenly gardens. Children often swing on the aerial roots of banyan trees. In some parts of India swings are commonly found in people's living rooms. In Lola-asana, even the yogi swings on his arms.

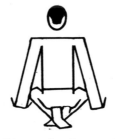 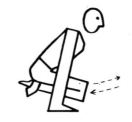 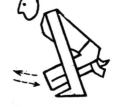

1. Sit on the floor with both legs bent back. Cross your ankles. Place your palms on the floor beside your legs. Keep your fingers pointing forward.

2. Straighten your elbows. Press your palms onto the floor and lift your legs off the floor. Swing back and forth. This is *Lola-asana.*

3. Then rest on the floor. Change the crossing of the legs. Repeat the pose.

BENEFITS

✿ Strengthens the fingers, wrists and arms.

✿ Tones the lower abdominal region.

DO

○ Raise your legs high off the floor.

DON'T

□ Don't look down.

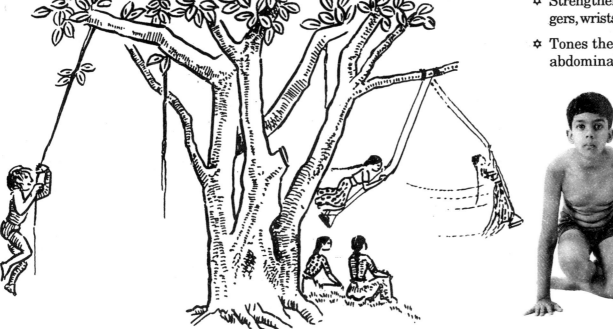

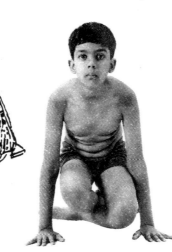

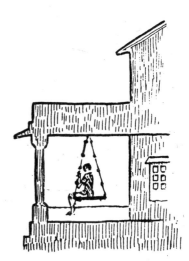

64. Nava-asana 10 to 15 counts

65. Ardha Nava-asana 10 to 15 counts

Nava means boat or ship. Ardha means half. The first pose resembles a boat with oars. The second is like a boat without oars.

Once there was a great flood. Heavy rains fell ceaselessly. The flood waters rose higher and higher till the whole earth was drowned. Only a few Himalayan peaks remained above the water.

A large wooden boat helped save Manu and various creatures and plants from destruction. Manu tied this boat to the horn of an enormous fish. The fish towed the boat towards a high peak which stood above the waters. Then Manu fastened his vessel to the peak. Since then this peak has been called Nav-bandhana Sringa, The-Peak-To-Which-The-Boat-Was-Fastened.

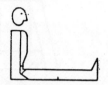

1. Sit in Danda-asana.

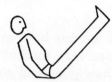

2. Lean back. Raise your legs till they are higher than your head.

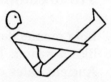

3. Extend your arms out in front of you. Keep your palms facing each other. This is *Nava-asana*.

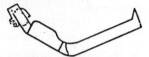

4. Then interlock your fingers behind your head. Lower your head and legs a little. This is *Ardha Nava-asana*.

DO

- Keep your legs as stiff as planks.
- Keep your arms as stiff as oars in Nava-asana.

DON'T

- Don't be like a sinking boat.

BENEFITS

- Strengthens the stomach muscles and the back.
- Tones the intestines, kidneys and liver.

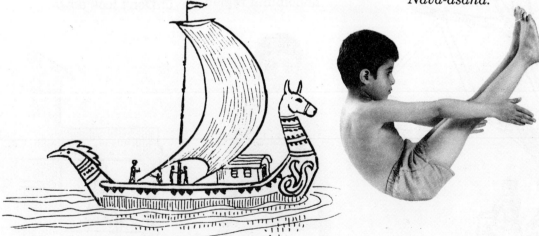

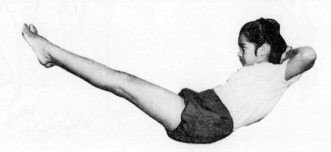

66. Urdhva Prasarita Pada-asana

10 to 15 counts at each pause

Urdhva means raised or upwards. Prasarita means stretched-out or spread and pada means foot.

Yoga is a precise subject. No movement should be done haphazardly. Be precise while you practice.

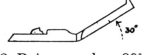

1. Lie on your back. Join your legs. Keep them poker stiff. Stretch your arms overhead with the palms facing up.

2. Raise your legs 30° off the floor. Pause.

3. Then raise your legs further to 60°. Pause.

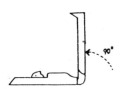

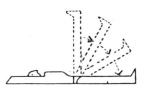

4. Then bring your legs to 90°, perpendicular to the floor. Pause. This is *Urdhva Prasarita Pada-asana.*

5. Then bring your legs down to 60°. Pause. Then to 30°. Pause. Then down to the floor.

DO

○ Keep your head, shoulders and arms on the floor.

○ Broaden the soles of your feet.

DON'T

☐ Don't crash land.

BENEFITS

✿ Trims the waist.

✿ Strengthens the organs of the abdomen.

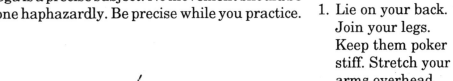

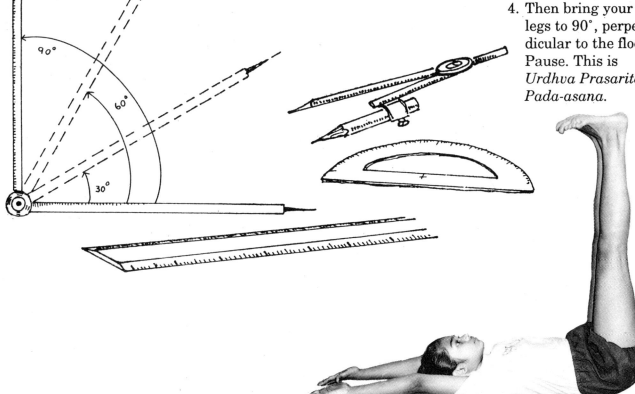

67 Bhuja-pida-asana

10 to 15 counts

Bhuja means arms or the trunk of an elephant. Pida means pressure. In this pose there is a lot of pressure on the arms, hence the name.

The second Pandava brother was the mighty Bhima. None could match his strength or courage. In the *Mahabharata* he is described as having arms like elephant trunks, legs like maces and a body as broad as a tree.

In his youth, Bhima was the scourge of his cousins, the Kauravas. He easily defeated them in sports and contests. Once, in a game, the five Pandava brothers were teamed against the hundred Kaurava brothers. Despite their numbers, the Kauravas were losing.

Unable to accept defeat, they began quarrelling with the Pandavas. Bhima was furious. He charged at the Kauravas to teach them a lesson!

The Kauravas fled and climbed up a large tree. Bhima embraced the tree trunk with his huge arms and shook the tree vigorously. The Kauravas dropped down like ripe fruit and ran for their lives.

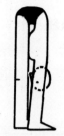

1. Stand in Uttana-asana with the feet about a foot apart.

2. Bend your knees. Insert your arms between your legs, and place your palms on the outer sides of your feet. Keep your fingers pointing forward.

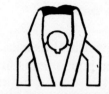

3. Rest the back of your knees on your upper arms. Gently raise both feet off the floor.

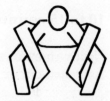

4. Cross your ankles. Look straight ahead. This is *Bhuja-pida-asana*. Then come down. Cross your ankles the other way, and repeat the pose.

DO
- Place your thighs high up on your arms.
- Lift your buttocks and feet high off the floor.

DON'T
- Don't look down.

BENEFITS
- Strengthens the wrists, arms, shoulders and abdomen.

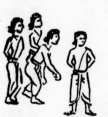
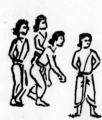
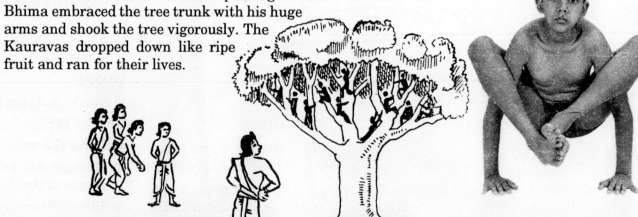

68. Ashta-vakra-asana

10 to 15 counts each side

Ashta means eight and vakra means bends. Ashta-vakra was a great sage. He was born with eight bends in his body. When Ashta-vakra was just a child of twelve he defeated Janaka's learned court scholar, Vandi, in a debate. In recognition of this great deed, King Janaka appointed the young Ashta-vakra as his teacher.

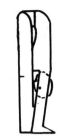

1. Stand in Uttana-asana with your feet about a foot apart.

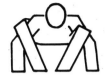

2. Bend your knees. Insert your right arm between your legs, and place your right hand on the outer side of your right foot. Then place your left hand on the floor on the outer side of your left foot. Do not take your left hand from between your legs.

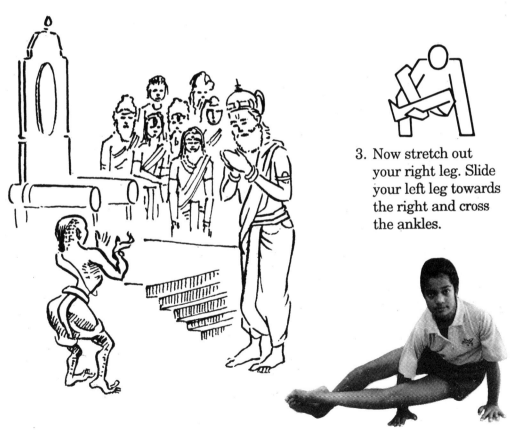

3. Now stretch out your right leg. Slide your left leg towards the right and cross the ankles.

4. Take the weight of your right leg on your right upper arm and raise your feet off the floor. Stretch your legs out sideways. This is *Ashta-vakra-asana.*

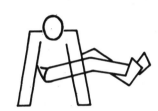

5. Then stand up. Now repeat the pose taking the weight of your left leg on your left arm.

DO

○ Grip your arms between your legs.

○ Keep your fingers well spread and pointing forward.

DON'T

☐ Don't slide down your arms.

BENEFITS

✿ Strengthens the arms and wrists.

✿ Strengthens the abdominal muscles.

69. Baka-asana

10 to 15 counts

Baka means a crane. Have you watched a crane waiting to catch its prey? It remains alert and still, concentrating its attention on a fish or a frog. So, keep your body steady and mind alert when you do Baka-asana.

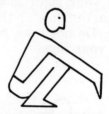

1. Squat.

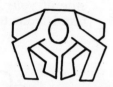

2. Spread your knees. Place your palms on the floor near your feet. Raise your hips. Raise your head. Rest your knees on your upper arms.

3. Sway your body forward. Raise your feet off the floor, one by one. Balance on your arms. This is *Baka-asana*. Then drop your feet to the floor and stand up.

DON'T

☐ Don't fall on your face, keep a blanket in front of you to serve as cushion.

DO

○ Join your toes.
○ Straighten your arms.
○ Keep your fingers well spread and pointing **forward**.

BENEFITS

✿ A challenging pose, **gives** strength and confidence.

✿ Improves concen**tration**.

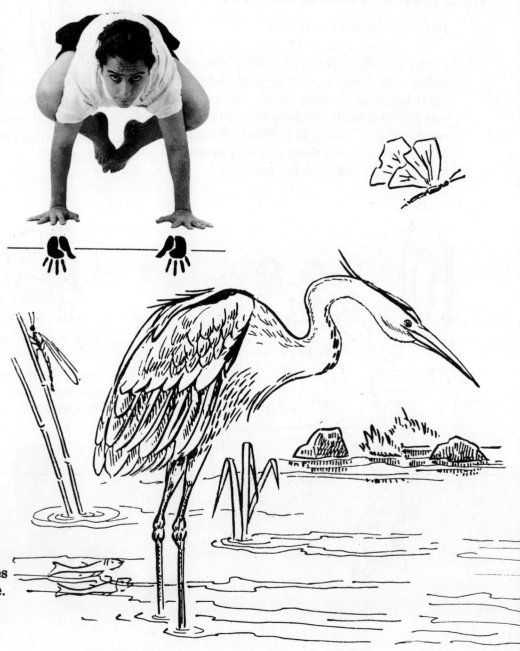

70 Bheka-asana

10 to 15 counts

Bheka means a frog. The sages of old not only observed the way the frog bent its legs, they also appreciated the frog's song. In classical Indian music the note dha, (which corresponds to A in the scale of western music), is inspired by the croaking of the frog.

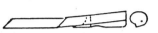

1. Lie on your stomach.

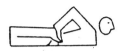

2. Bend your knees. Place your palms on your feet. Turn your wrist, so that your fingers point in the same direction as your toes.

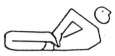

3. Press your feet downwards and raise your chest off the floor. Look up. This is *Bheka-asana*.

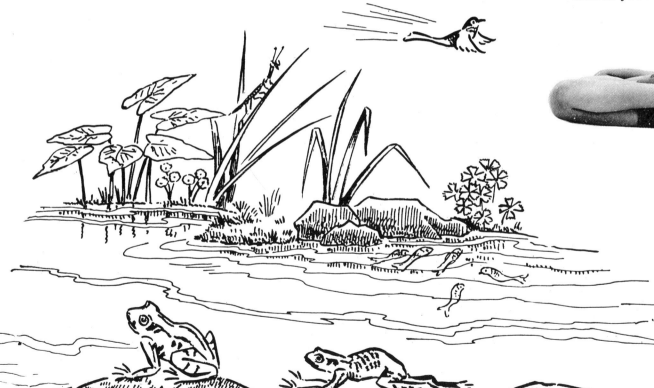

DO
○ Bend your legs like a frog.

DON'T
☐ Don't turn your fingers sideways.

BENEFITS
✿ Strengthens and corrects defects in the knees.

✿ Strengthens the ankles.

✿ Improves flat feet.

71. Nakra-asana

repeat several times

Nakra means a crocodile. About thirteen hundred years ago there lived a great and learned sage named Shankara. He was born in the Malabar region of South India. When he was a boy he wished to renounce the world and become a sanyasi. His mother did not permit this and instead arranged a marriage for him.

One day while Shankara and his mother were bathing in the river, a crocodile grabbed Shankara's foot. Thinking that his end had come, he begged his mother, "Please, Mother, now grant me my wish to become a sanyasi so I may die content."

His mother immediately consented. All of a sudden the crocodile released Shankara.

Shankara became a sanyasi. He travelled the length and breadth of **India** spreading the light of wisdom. He established many monasteries and temples.

BENEFITS

✿ Develops the wrists and arms.

✿ Makes you strong.

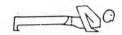

1. Do Chatur-anga Danda-asana.

DO

○ Lunge forward like a crocodile catching its prey.

○ Raise your whole body off the floor while leaping.

DON'T

☐ Don't rest your thighs on the floor.

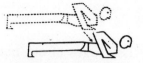

2. Leap forward. Land in Chatur-anga Danda-asana. Again leap forward. Repeat several times.

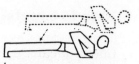

3. Then move backwards in leaps. Land in Chaturanga Danda-asana each time. This is *Nakra-asana.*

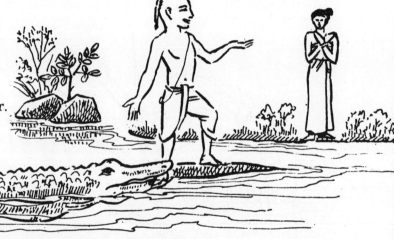

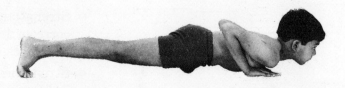

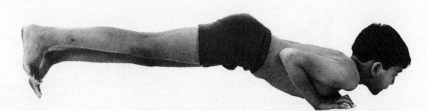

72. Chakra-asana

Repeat several times

Chakra means wheel or discus. The Sudarshana Chakra, Lord Vishnu's celestial discus, is considered the most powerful weapon anywhere. Fiery-golden in colour, its cutting edges are never dull. Its tremendous speed and great power create terror amongst the enemies of the gods.

There is an interesting tale of how the Sudarshana Chakra was wrought. The Sun God's wife couldn't bear her husband's intense radiance. She complained to her father, Vishva-karma, the artisan of the gods.

Vishva-karma then ground the sun on his grinding machine and reduced its intensity by one-eighth. Then, from the leftover blazing bits, Vishva-karma fashioned fiery weapons for the gods. The Sudarshana Chakra, Lord Shiva's trident and Lord Kartikeya's lance were all made from these solar fragments.

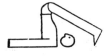

1. Do Hala-asana.

2. Bend your knees. Place your palms under your shoulders. Keep your fingers pointing away from your feet.

3 Press your palms onto the floor. Raise your neck and shoulders off the floor and do a reverse somersault! Roll over onto your knees. This is *Chakra-asana*.

DO
- Roll over quickly.

DON'T
- Don't tumble sideways.

BENEFITS
- Makes the body light and flexible

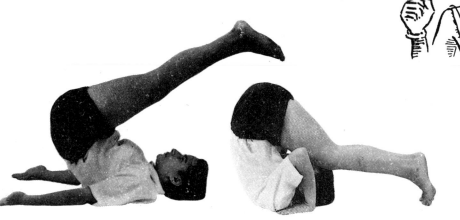

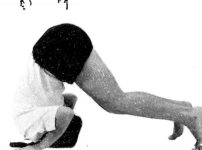

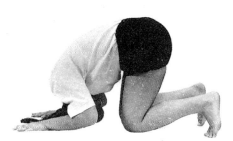

73. Akarna Dhanur-asana

10 to 15 counts

Karna means the ear and the prefix "A" means near. Dhanu means a bow. This pose resembles an archer drawing his bow.

Karna, the son of Surya, the Sun God, was a renowned archer. He was called Karna because he was born with shining rings in his ears. These earings and a suit of armour were divine gifts from his father. As long as Karna wore these, he would remain invicible in battle!

Karna's great rival was his half-brother, the illustrious archer Arjuna. Arjuna's father, Lord Indra, dreaded that Karna might, one day, defeat and kill Arjuna. Indra therefore played a trick on Karna. Disguised as a poor brahmin, Indra approached Karna.

"O noble warrior," he said, " grant me a wish."

"Ask and you shall have whatever you want," replied Karna, who was well known for his generosity.

"Give me your earings and armour," asked the crafty Indra.

Though Karna knew that he would lose his magic protection he unhesitatingly parted with his divine possessions.

Later, during the Mahabharata war, in one of the greatest battles fought in the history of archery, Karna was defeated and killed by Arjuna.

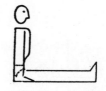

1. Sit in Danda-asana.

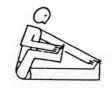

2. Hook your left big toe with your left index and middle fingers.

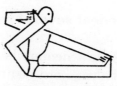

3. Then hook your right big toe with your right index and middle fingers. Pull your right foot to your right ear. This is *Akarna Dhanur-asana*. Then do this pose on the other side.

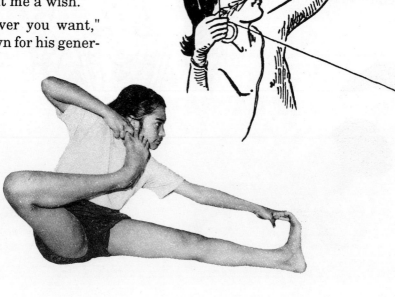

DO

○ Draw your bent leg back like an archer draws his bow string.

DON'T

☐ Don't bring your ear to your foot, bring your foot to your ear.

BENEFITS

✿ Keeps the numerous joints of the body strong and flexible.

74. Ananta-asana

10 to 15 counts each side

Ananta means endless or infinite. Lord Vishnu is sometimes called Ananta. When the world ends, Lord Vishnu lies down to rest on the coiled body of an enormous, thousand-hooded serpent. The serpent is also called Ananta.

After Lord Vishnu has rested for many aeons, a lotus stem sprouts from his navel. From the heart of this lotus Lord Brahma is born. Brahma then recreates the universe.

This pose represents Lord Vishnu resting on the snake, Ananta.

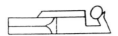

1 Lie on your left side. Support your head with your left hand. Keep both legs straight.

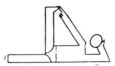

2. Bend your right leg. Hook your right big toe with your right middle and index fingers. Then raise your right leg vertically. This is *Ananta-asana*.

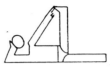

3. Then roll over onto your right side. Now do the pose with your left leg stretched vertically.

DO

○ Keep the side of your body on a straight line when you lie down.

○ Tighten the muscles of your thighs and buttocks.

DON'T

☐ Don't bend your knees.

BENEFITS

✿ Strengthens the back muscles.

✿ Makes the hamstrings elastic.

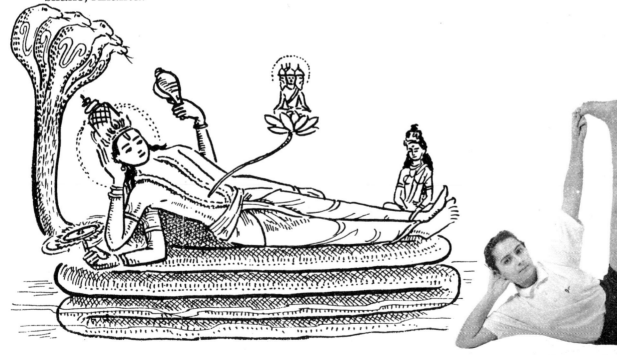

75. Shava-asana

2 to 5 minutes

Shava means a dead body. There once lived a beautiful and virtuous princess named Savitri. She chose a young prince named Satyavan for her husband. Though he was a prince, Satyavan lived in a hermitage with his parents. His father, the exiled king of Salaya, was blind.

Savitri married Satyavan although she knew that he was fated to die within one year of their marriage. She fasted and prayed to prepare herself for this fateful event. On the appointed day, when Satyavan went to cut wood in the forest, Savitri accompanied him. While chopping wood Satyavan's head began to hurt. Savitri laid her husband's head on her lap and soothed him.

While sitting thus in the shade of a large tree, Savitri saw Yama, the God of Death, approaching them. Humbly she folded her palms to him, "Why have you come?" she asked.

"I have come to take Satyavan's soul to the land of the dead," said Yama. So saying, he ensnared Satyavan's soul in his noose and began to walk away.

The courageous Savitri left Satyavan's dead body under the tree and hurriedly followed the God of Death.

"Why are you following me, fair maid?" asked Yama. "Your husband's time has come. Nothing can save him."

Savitri did not stop. "I see you are a brave and devoted lady," said the God of Death. "Ask for a boon other than your husband's life."

"Give my father-in-law back his sight," asked Savitri.

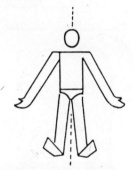

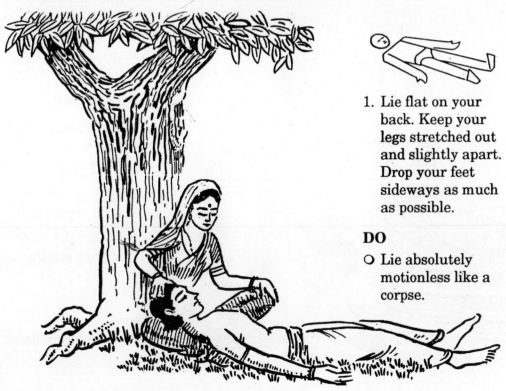

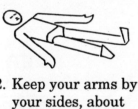

1. Lie flat on your back. Keep your **legs** stretched out and slightly apart. Drop your feet sideways as much as possible.

DO
- Lie absolutely motionless like a corpse.

2. Keep your arms by your sides, about 50° away from the chest. Keep your palms turned up.

- Loosen every part of your body: toes, fingers, thighs, arms, stomach, throat, lips, cheeks, forehead.

DON'T
- Don't lie crooked.
- Don't tilt your head.

3. Close your eyes. Keep your chin pointing towards your chest. Breathe normally. Relax. This is *Shava-asana*.

BENEFITS
- Relaxes the nerves and the brain.
- Removes fatigue.
- Teaches concentration.
- Calms the emotions.

"So be it. Now Savitri, go back. This path is not for mortals."

Savitri still followed Yama. Seeing this, Yama said, "For your perseverance ask for another boon."

"Let my father-in-law regain his kingdom," prayed Savitri.

"Granted," said Yama, "and now you must turn back."

The devoted and virtuous Savitri did not turn back. Yama was perplexed. Once again he offered her a boon.

"My father has no sons," said Savitri. "Grant him a hundred sons."

"This too I grant. Now return immediately, Savitri. This path is dark and dangerous."

Undaunted, Savitri walked on behind Yama. Touched by her devotion, Yama granted her one last boon.

"Grant me many children," asked Savitri.

"Granted," replied Yama.

"But how can I have children without my husband," pleaded Savitri. "You must restore my husband to life."

Bound by his word Yama restored Satyavan to life.

Savitri rushed back and found Satyavan stirring. She helped him back to the hermitage. Satyavan's father could see when they returned. The next morning a delegation of courtiers invited the exiled king to return and govern his kingdom. Satyavan became the heir to the throne. Over the years Savitri's father had many sons. Savitri and Satyavan, also had many children and lived a long and happy life.

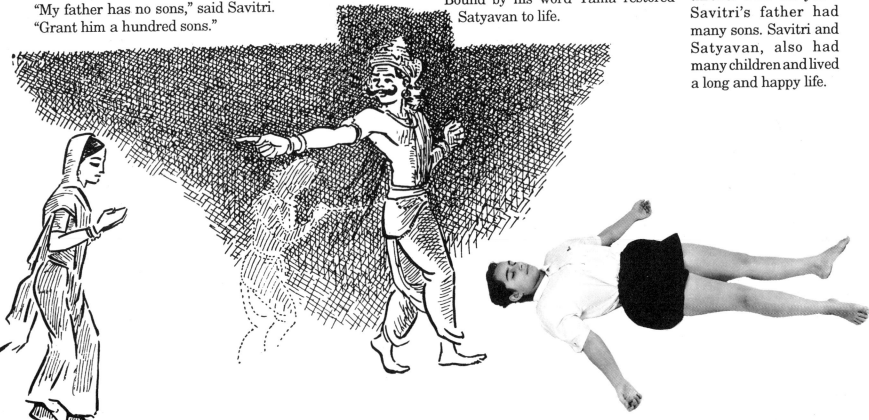

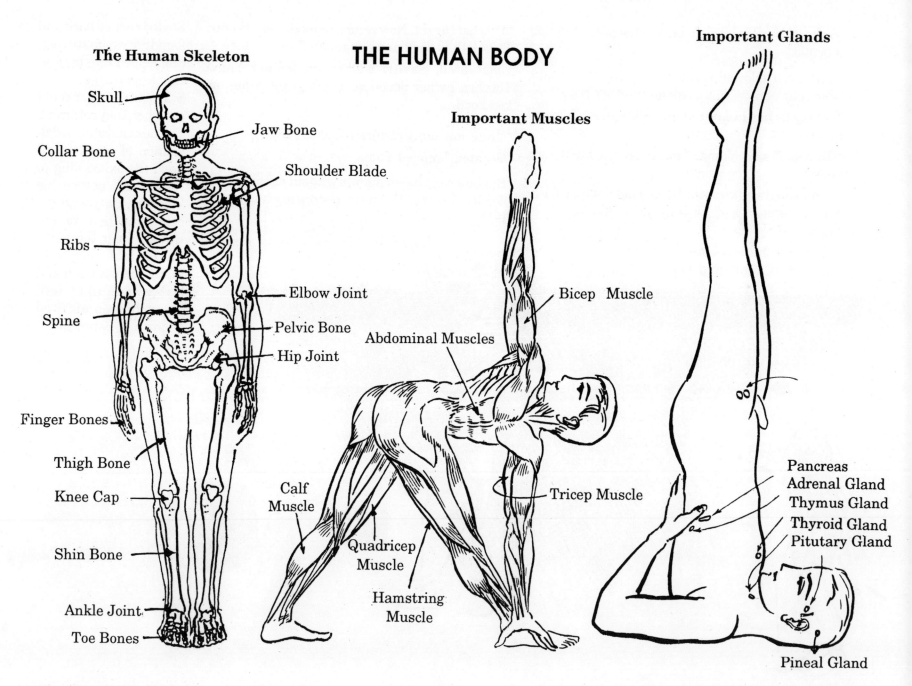

THE HUMAN BODY

The Human Skeleton

Skull

Jaw Bone

Collar Bone

Shoulder Blade

Ribs

Elbow Joint

Spine

Pelvic Bone

Hip Joint

Finger Bones

Thigh Bone

Knee Cap

Shin Bone

Ankle Joint

Toe Bones

Important Muscles

Bicep Muscle

Abdominal Muscles

Tricep Muscle

Calf Muscle

Quadricep Muscle

Hamstring Muscle

Important Glands

Pancreas
Adrenal Gland
Thymus Gland
Thyroid Gland
Pitutary Gland

Pineal Gland

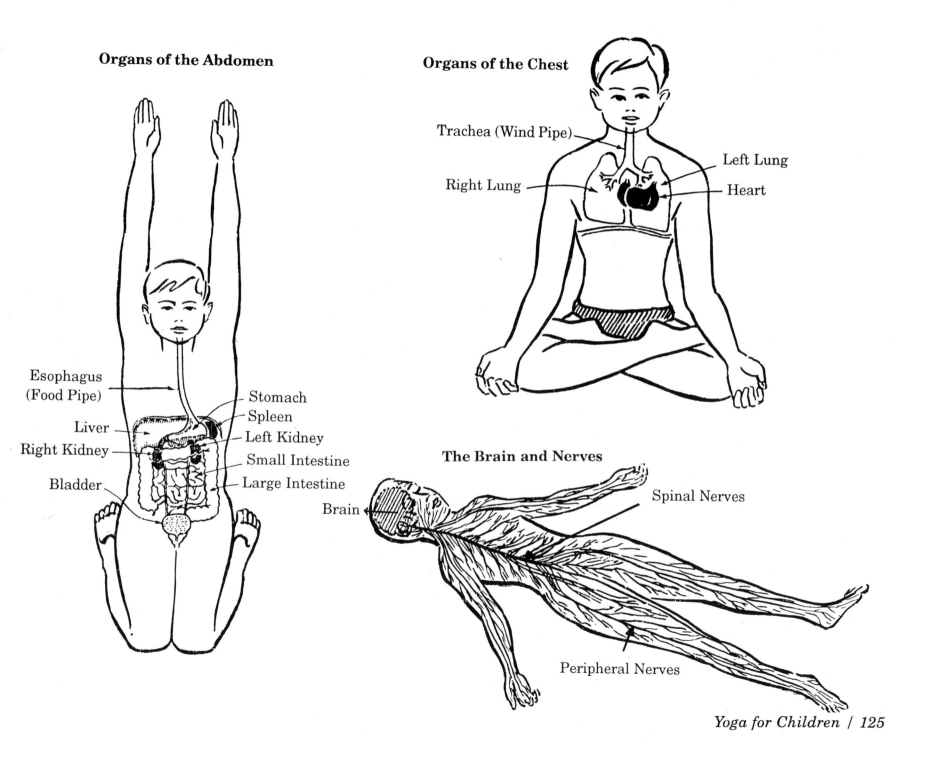

Organs of the Abdomen

Esophagus
(Food Pipe)

Liver

Right Kidney

Bladder

Stomach

Spleen

Left Kidney

Small Intestine

Large Intestine

Organs of the Chest

Trachea (Wind Pipe)

Right Lung

Left Lung

Heart

The Brain and Nerves

Brain

Spinal Nerves

Peripheral Nerves

> - *The practice routines are illustrated in the order in which they have to be practiced.*
> - *Warm up well before you begin your practice.*
> - *Repeat each difficult asana two or three times.*
> - *Read the important DOs and Don'ts on page nos. 32-33.*

Practices Routines

COURSE I   Practice time: 20-25 minutes

- Course I is for beginners. Practice six days a week and rest on Sundays. Move on to Course II as soon as you can easily do the asanas of Course I.

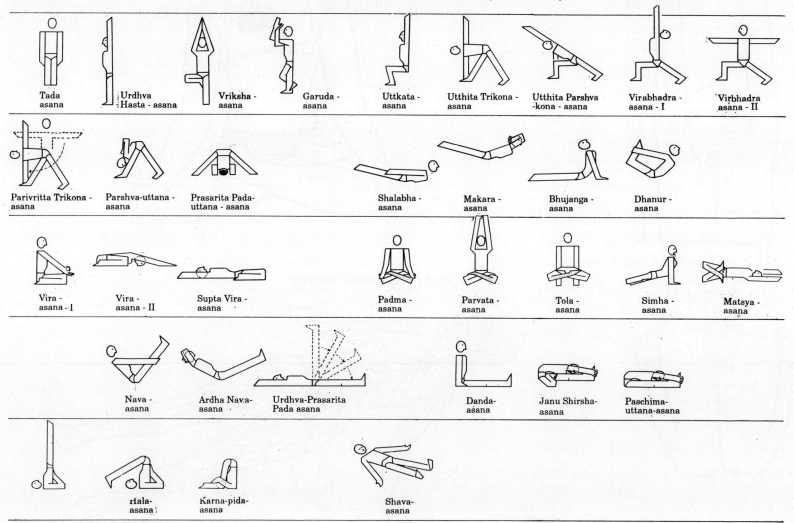

| Tada asana | Urdhva Hasta - asana | Vriksha - asana | Garuda - asana | Uttkata - asana | Utthita Trikona - asana | Utthita Parshva -kona - asana | Virabhadra - asana - I | Virbhadra asana - II |

| Parivritta Trikona - asana | Parshva-uttana - asana | Prasarita Pada-uttana - asana | | Shalabha - asana | Makara - asana | Bhujanga - asana | Dhanur - asana |

| Vira - asana - I | Vira - asana - II | Supta Vira - asana | | Padma - asana | Parvata - asana | Tola - asana | Simha - asana | Matsya - asana |

| Nava - asana | Ardha Nava - asana | Urdhva-Prasarita Pada asana | | Danda - asana | Janu Shirsha - asana | Paschima- uttana-asana |

| Hala - asana | Karna-pida- asana | Shava - asana |

- Course II has been divided into two parts i.e. Day 1 and Day 2. On Mondays, Wednesdays and Fridays practice the asanas of Day 1. On Tuesdays, Thursdays and Saturdays practice the asanas of Day 2. Rest on Sundays.

- After some days ask your teacher to suggest new asanas and challenging movements which can fit into this course.

COURSE II, Day-1 Practice time: 30 to 35 minutes

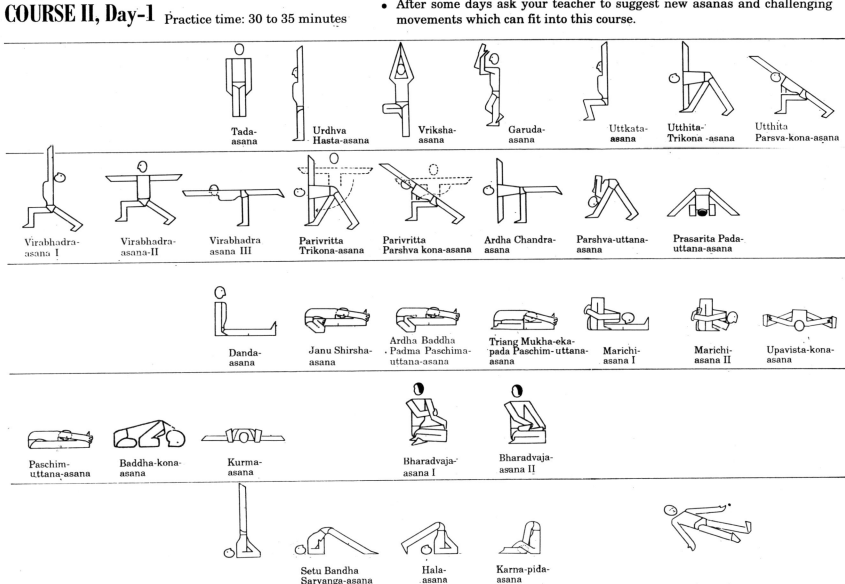

Tada-asana

Urdhva Hasta-asana

Vriksha-asana

Garuda-asana

Uttkata-asana

Utthita Trikona-asana

Utthita Parsva-kona-asana

Virabhadra-asana I

Virabhadra-asana-II

Virabhadra-asana III

Parivritta Trikona-asana

Parivritta Parshva kona-asana

Ardha Chandra-asana

Parshva-uttana-asana

Prasarita Pada-uttana-asana

Danda-asana

Janu Shirsha-asana

Ardha Baddha Padma Paschima-uttana-asana

Triang Mukha-eka-pada Paschim-uttana-asana

Marichi-asana I

Marichi-asana II

Upavista-kona-asana

Paschim-uttana-asana

Baddha-kona-asana

Kurma-asana

Bharadvaja-asana I

Bharadvaja-asana II

Setu Bandha Sarvanga-asana

Hala-asana

Karna-pida-asana

COURSE II, Day-2

• After several weeks, when you can do the asanas of Course II easily, move on to Course III.

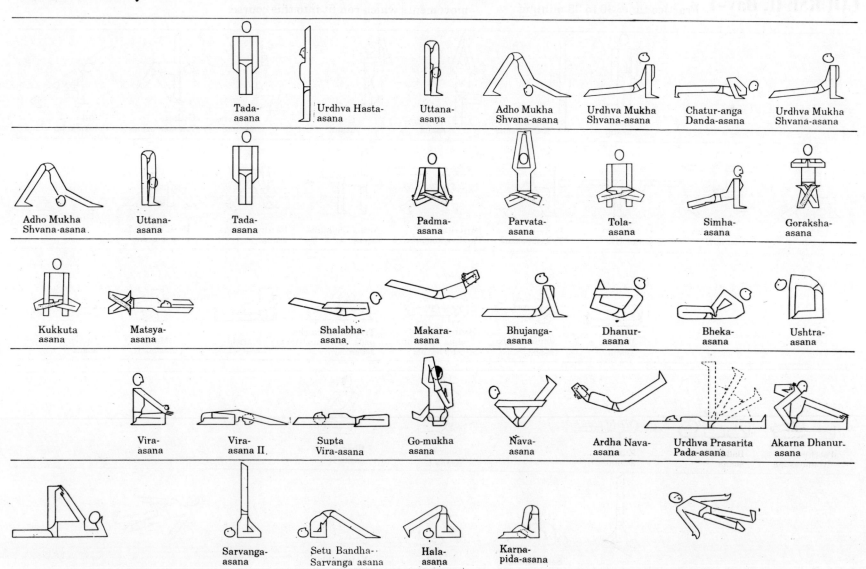

| Tada-asana | Urdhva Hasta-asana | Uttana-asana | Adho Mukha Shvana-asana | Urdhva Mukha Shvana-asana | Chatur-anga Danda-asana | Urdhva Mukha Shvana-asana |

| Adho Mukha Shvana-asana | Uttana-asana | Tada-asana | Padma-asana | Parvata-asana | Tola-asana | Simha-asana | Goraksha-asana |

| Kukkuta asana | Matsya-asana | Shalabha-asana | Makara-asana | Bhujanga-asana | Dhanur-asana | Bheka-asana | Ushtra-asana |

| Vira-asana | Vira-asana II | Supta Vira-asana | Go-mukha asana | Nava-asana | Ardha Nava-asana | Urdhva Prasarita Pada-asana | Akarna Dhanur-asana |

| Sarvanga-asana | Setu Bandha-Sarvanga asana | Hala-asana | Karna-pida-asana |

- Course III includes all 75 asanas explained in this book, and the course has been divided into three parts. On Mondays and Thursdays do the asanas of Day 1. On Tuesdays and Fridays do the asanas of Day 2. On Wednesdays and Saturdays do the asanas of Day 3. Rest on Sundays.

COURSE III, Day-1

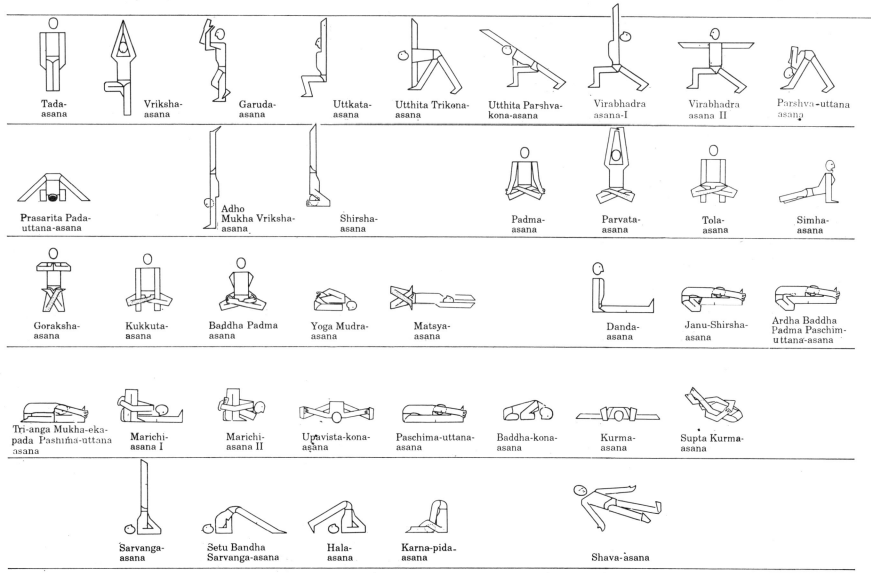

Tada-asana	Vriksha-asana	Garuda-asana	Uttkata-asana	Utthita Trikona-asana	Utthita Parshva-kona-asana	Virabhadra asana-I	Virabhadra asana II	Parshva-uttana asana
Prasarita Pada-uttana-asana		Adho Mukha Vriksha-asana	Shirsha-asana		Padma-asana	Parvata-asana	Tola-asana	Simha-asana
Goraksha-asana	Kukkuta-asana	Baddha Padma asana	Yoga Mudra-asana	Matsya-asana		Danda-asana	Janu-Shirsha-asana	Ardha Baddha Padma Paschim-uttana-asana
Tri-anga Mukha-eka-pada Pashima-uttana asana	Marichi-asana I	Marichi-asana II	Upavista-kona-asana	Paschima-uttana-asana	Baddha-kona-asana	Kurma-asana	Supta Kurma-asana	
Sarvanga-asana	Setu Bandha Sarvanga-asana	Hala-asana	Karna-pida-asana		Shava-asana			

COURSE III, Day-2

Practice time 35 to 45 minutes

• Ask to your teacher to suggest new asanas and challenging movements which can be added to your practice.

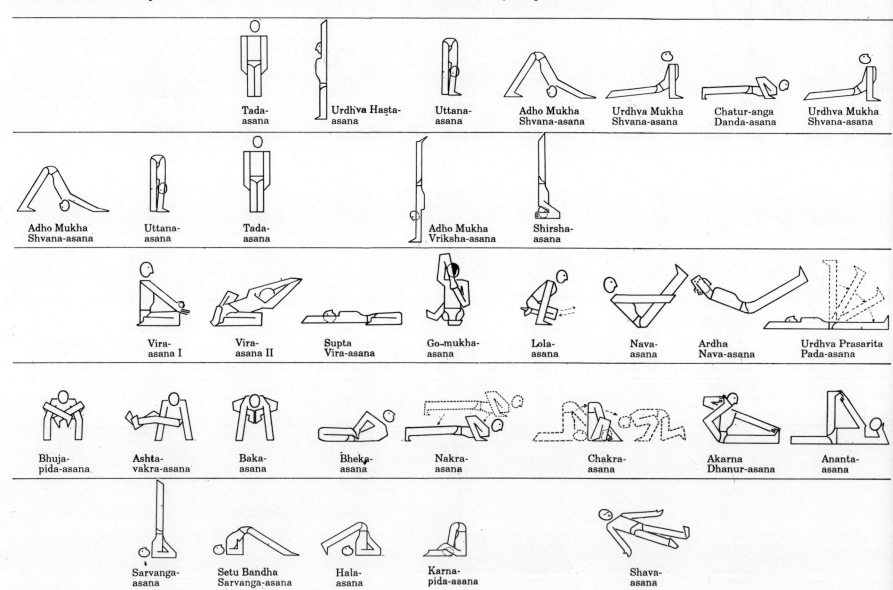

Tada-asana

Urdhva Hasta-asana

Uttana-asana

Adho Mukha Shvana-asana

Urdhva Mukha Shvana-asana

Chatur-anga Danda-asana

Urdhva Mukha Shvana-asana

Adho Mukha Shvana-asana

Uttana-asana

Tada-asana

Adho Mukha Vriksha-asana

Shirsha-asana

Vira-asana I

Vira-asana II

Supta Vira-asana

Go-mukha-asana

Lola-asana

Nava-asana

Ardha Nava-asana

Urdhva Prasarita Pada-asana

Bhuja-pida-asana

Ashta-vakra-asana

Baka-asana

Bheka-asana

Nakra-asana

Chakra-asana

Akarna Dhanur-asana

Ananta-asana

Sarvanga-asana

Setu Bandha Sarvanga-asana

Hala-asana

Karna-pida-asana

Shava-asana

OURSE III, Day 3

Practice time: 35 to 45 minutes

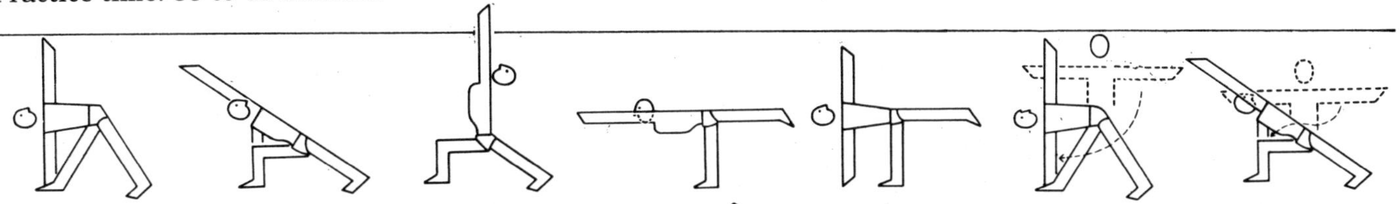

Utthita Trikona-asana | Utthita Parshva-kona-asana | Virabhadra-asana I | Virabhadra-asana III | Ardha Chandra-asana | Parivritta Trikona-asana | Parivritta Parshva-kona-asana

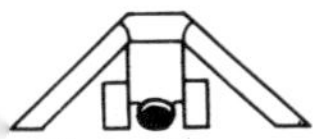

Prasarita Pada-uttana-asana

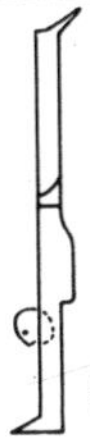

Adho Mukha Vriksha-asana

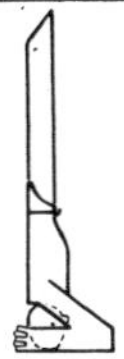

Shirsha-asana

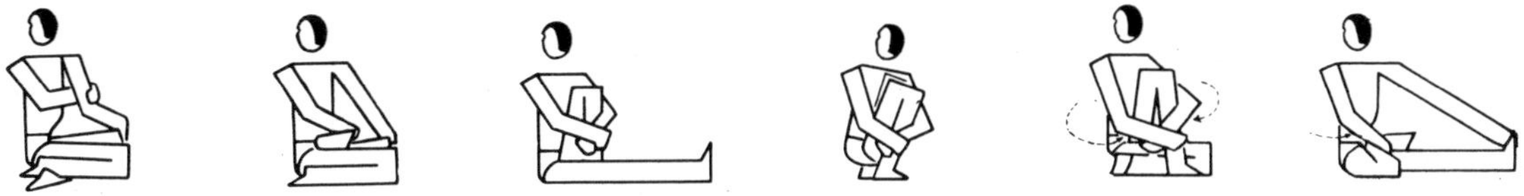

Bharadvaja-asana I | Bharadvaja-asana II | Marichi-asana III | Pasha-asana | Ardha Matsyendra-asana I | Ardha Matsyendra-asana II

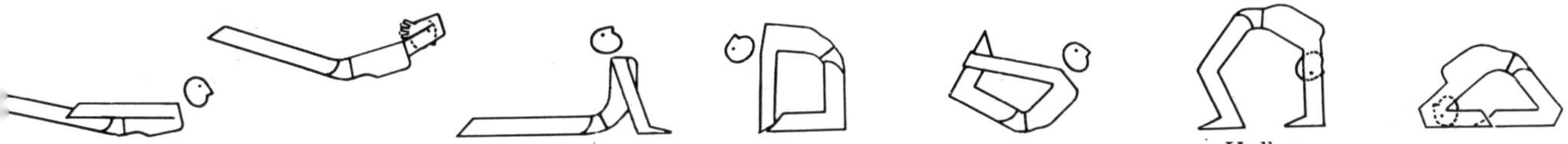

Shalabha-asana | Makara-asana | Bhujanga-asana | Ushtra-asana | Dhanur-asana | Urdhva Dhanur-asana | Kapota-asana

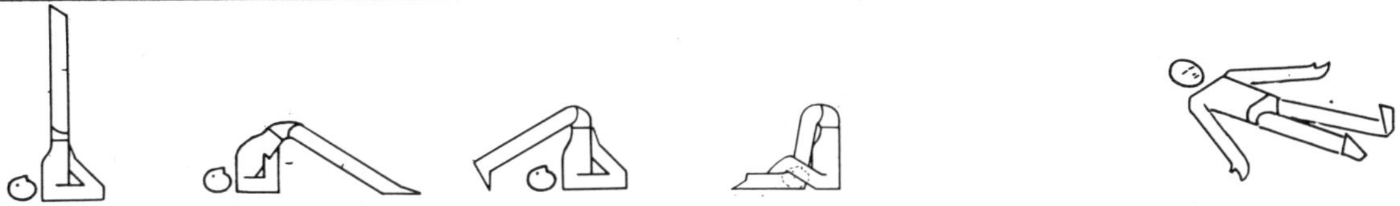

Sarvanga-asana | Setu Bandha Sarvanga-asana | Hala-asana | Karna-Pida-asana | Shava-asana

THE YOGA ASANA CHART

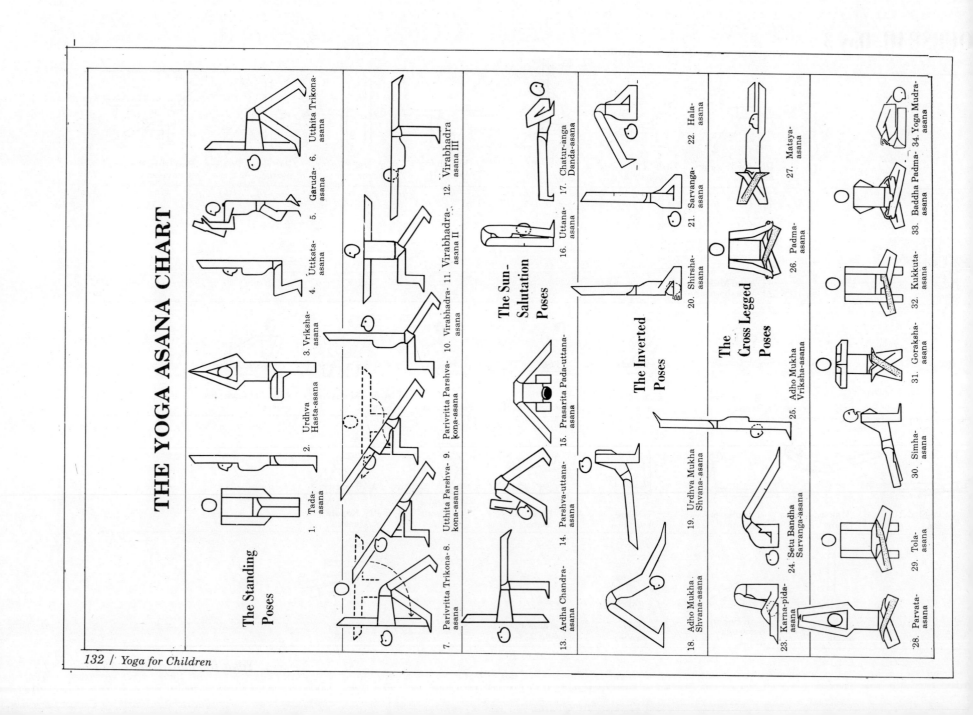

The Standing Poses

1. Tada-asana
2. Urdhva Hasta-asana
3. Vriksha-asana
4. Utkkata-asana
5. Garuda-asana
6. Utthita Trikona-asana
7. Parivritta Trikona-asana
8. Utthita Parshva-kona-asana
9. Parivritta Parshva-kona-asana
10. Virabhadra-asana
11. Virabhadra-asana II
12. Virabhadra-asana III
13. Ardha Chandra-asana
14. Parshva-uttana-asana
15. Prasarita Pada-uttana-asana

The Sun-Salutation Poses

16. Uttana-asana
17. Chatur-anga Danda-asana
18. Adho Mukha Shvana-asana
19. Urdhva Mukha Shvana-asana

The Inverted Poses

20. Shirsha-asana
21. Sarvanga-asana
22. Hala-asana
23. Karna-pida-asana
24. Setu Bandha Sarvanga-asana
25. Adho Mukha Vriksha-asana

The Cross Legged Poses

26. Padma-asana
27. Matsya-asana
28. Parvata-asana
29. Tola-asana
30. Simha-asana
31. Goraksha-asana
32. Kukkuta-asana
33. Baddha Padma-asana
34. Yoga Mudra-asana

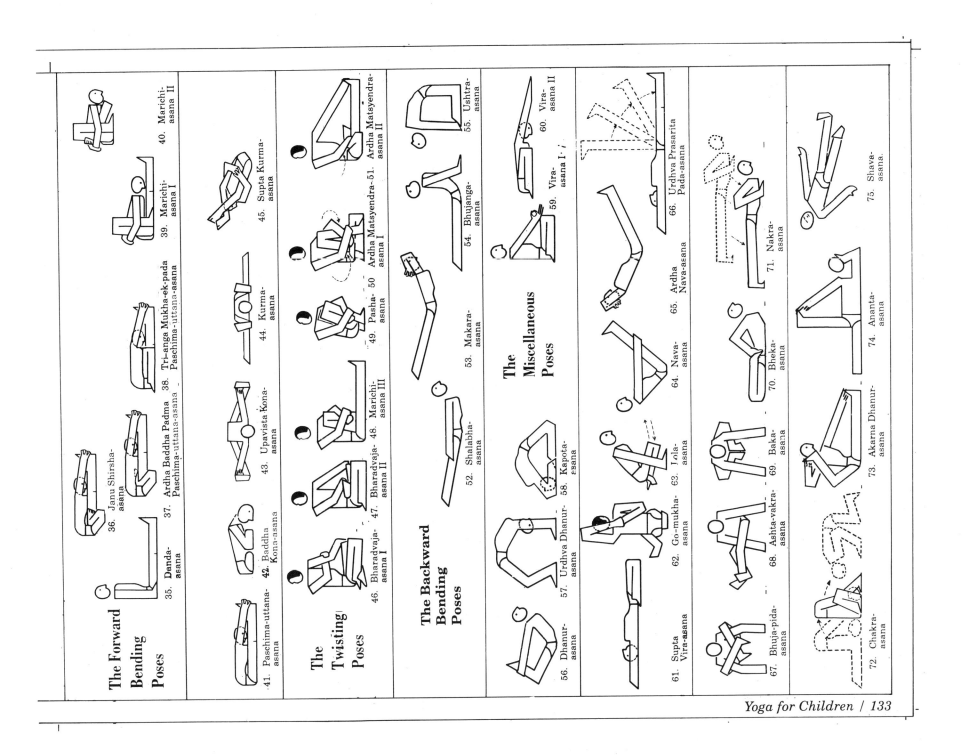

The Forward Bending Poses

35. Danda-asana
36. Janu Shirsha-asana
37. Ardha Baddha Padma Paschima-uttana-asana
38. Tri-anga Mukha-ek-pada Paschima-uttana-asana
39. Marichi-asana I
40. Marichi-asana II
41. Paschima-uttana-asana
42. Baddha Kona-asana
43. Upavista Kona-asana
44. Kurma-asana
45. Supta Kurma-asana

The Twisting Poses

46. Bharadvaja-asana I
47. Bharadvaja-asana II
48. Marichi-asana III
49. Pasha-asana
50. Ardha Matsyendra-asana I
51. Ardha Matsyendra-asana II

The Backward Bending Poses

52. Shalabha-asana
53. Makara-asana
54. Bhujanga-asana
55. Ushtra-asana
56. Dhanur-asana
57. Urdhva Dhanur-asana
58. Kapota-asana
59. Vira-asana I
60. Vira-asana II

The Miscellaneous Poses

61. Supta Vira-asana
62. Go-mukha-asana
63. Lola-asana
64. Nava-asana
65. Ardha Nava-asana
66. Urdhva Prasarita Pada-asana
67. Bhuja-pida-asana
68. Ashta-vakra-asana
69. Baka-asana
70. Bheka-asana
71. Nakra-asana
72. Chakra-asana
73. Akarna Dhanur-asana
74. Ananta-asana
75. Shava-asana.

A Manual for
Parents and Teachers

A Note to the Reader

This manual has been written to complement **Yoga for Children**. We hope that it will be useful to teachers and parents in guiding, motivating and assisting their children to practice Yoga.

Classical Sanskrit words, including names of asanas, have been broken down into simpler forms which make for easy reading and pronunciation. Diacritical marks have not been used as children find these difficult to understand.

1. Stretch Like a Dog

Stretch like a dog, bend your legs like a frog...sit straight as a rod...lunge like a crocodile...be tall as a mountain... withdraw your limbs like a sleeping turtle...don't be like a sunken boat....

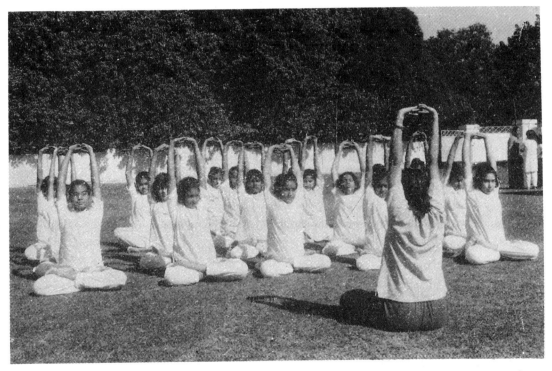

We found ourselves using many such metaphors while exhorting children to attain or improve a pose during a Yoga class. It was from these metaphors that this book was conceived. Yoga for children is certainly one way to ensure that our children grow up healthy and happy.

Of the many aspects of Yoga, yama, niyama and asana are relevant for children. While the principles yama and niyama reinforce the universal values such as truth, non-violence, cleanliness and contentment, the asanas help a growing child develop physically, emotionally and psychologically. In this way Yoga is a necessary complement to formal education. By practicing this wonderful science and art children can blossom into healthy, and well balanced men and women with strong bodies, clear minds and pure hearts.

In this endeavor the role of the Yoga teacher is crucial. The teacher must understand the nature of children and be sensitive to the moods and needs of the growing child. Children are creative by nature. They are expressive, outgoing and exuberant. They are courageous and curious and also sincere and devout. They are positive in nature. They are quick and agile and love variety and novelty.

Yoga-asanas are well suited for children. They are imaginative and unique. Asanas can be demonstrated, imitated and adapted. The asanas are dynamic, intense and challenging. They help a child to develop willpower, and sensitivity and provide children a means to learn about themselves through a wide range of body movements.

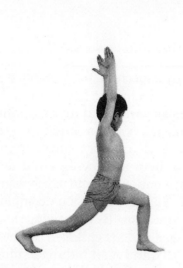
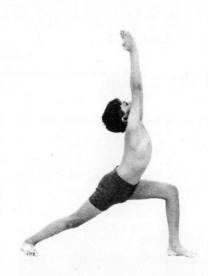
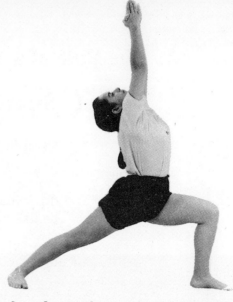

Childhood is a process of change, from fragility to strength, from immaturity to maturity, from simplicity to complexity. Accordingly, the approach for the six year old, the ten year old and the sixteen year old must vary greatly.

Little children should begin to learn the asanas playfully. They lack muscular strength and they must not be forced. They love animals and nature and also the poses inspired by these.

Ten year old children are co-operative and delight in Yoga. They are agile but no longer so fragile. They love to try out a wide range of movements.

Pubescent children pose a challenge to the teacher. They are in a state of physical upheaval and psychological turmoil. The Yoga teacher should teach them the asanas which help them to overcome their awkwardness and gain equilibrium.

Adolescents aged sixteen to eighteen are stronger, more energetic and can grasp some of the nuances in the asanas. They can be taught more techniques and the teacher must demand more precision from them. For these teen-agers both the intensity and the duration of the asanas can be increased.

Despite these differences all children have many things in common. They love dynamic movements with quick changes. Speed and variety are essential to keep their interest in the Yoga-asanas. They love expressive and outgoing asanas like the backward-bending poses and the head-stand. Though children are courageous they are not foolhardy. They are also physically and emotionally resilient.

Yoga teachers should avoid teaching children the advanced or esoteric aspects of Yoga such as meditation, pranayama, bandhas and shatkriyas These practices are contrary to the nature of children. While Yoga theory can and should be introduced to older children, it should be secondary to the practice of asanas and should be taught as informally as possible.

The most suitable place to introduce Yoga to children is in schools. A teacher would be well advised to group children of approximately the same age in a Yoga class as they need to be taught according to their capacities and inclinations. Teaching the asanas step by step and using counts to synchronize the children's movements is a particularly useful technique.

A Yoga teacher must therefore inspire children to practice the Yoga-asanas so that children love to stretch like dogs and bend their legs like frogs.

2. The Role of a Yoga Teacher

By Geeta Iyengar

The role of the Yoga teacher is of foremost importance if Yoga is to be successfully introduced to children. The Yoga teacher must be able to arouse curiosity in the pupils and create in them a desire to learn. He or she must inspire and enthuse the children and should be cheerful in the class.

A Yoga teacher must, therefore, have physical agility and mental sharpness. The teacher should be a keen practitioner of Yoga. He should be able to do the asanas along with the children and not just make demands of them and command them to do the poses. The teacher's subjective involvement is essential as children primarily learn by seeing and imitating. Children's eyes catch the movement quickly while they detest lengthy explanations. In any case, quick and agile movements cannot be explained, they have to be imparted directly. The teacher should also be quick to catch the mistakes of the pupils. He must correct and adjust their poses.

Children need a lot of variety and novelty. They don't want to repeat the same thing again and again. If they are forced to bring perfection, they do not like it; it has to be introduced gradually. Slow classes are boring and dissipate the child's energy. I noticed that some teachers were going too slow and restricting the child's capacity. Instead the teacher should be fast and teach dynamic movements. This will attract children who are otherwise easily distracted. Children are bursting with energy. One should not limit or hamper it.

Here I want to point out that though some teachers say that only simple asanas ought to be taught to children this strategy won't work for long. Though initially children do not hesitate to perform simple and soft movements, after a few turns they themselves show a reluctuance to do such easy movements. They realize that though they are painless they are effectless. Children have a potential strength and courage which the teacher must draw out.

The teacher should keep in mind that children have a tremendous defensive strength. Therefore, injuries do not occur easily. If something goes wrong while performing the asanas, children stop doing immediately without being told to do so. They have a self-guarding and self-protecting intelligence. It is inherent at this age. They are not adamant like elders though they are very courageous.

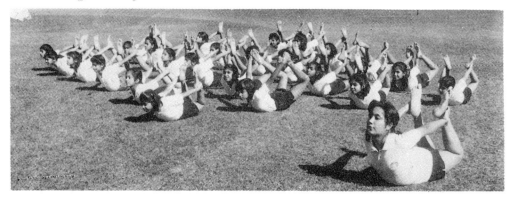

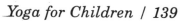

3. Little Children

By Geeta Iyengar

Teachers and parents are often uncertain about the age at which children should commence Yoga practice. Children aged eight years and above are fit to practice Yoga. Children between the ages of five and eight can also do some asanas. However, they are too young to practice Yoga formally. While the static poses do not suit these children, they don't have the capacity to do many dynamic movements either. It is true that these little children are very supple and elastic. However, at this tender age their suppleness, vibrancy and elasticity should not be taxed. Little children lack muscular strength. Furthermore, a Yoga class of 20 or 25 minutes duration becomes too long for them. Little children should be permitted to playfully and casually learn a few postures. It would be a misguided effort to make Yoga compulsory for them. Little children should be permitted to grow up naturally. The discipline should not be imposed too early.

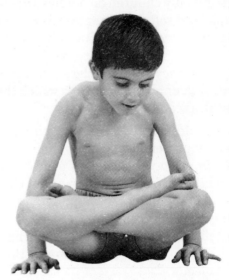

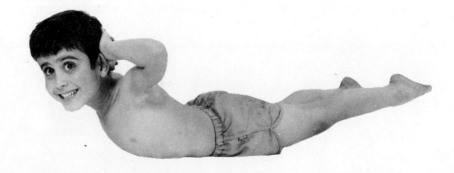

4. Adolescents

Adolescence is the stage between childhood and maturity roughly between the ages twelve and twenty. During this period, around the age of fourteen, a child reaches puberty, reproductive capability. Remarkable biological changes occur in spurts, often outstripping psychological growth. In particular, the endocrinal glands undergo important changes and their enhanced functioning stimulates new patterns of growth and evolution. Yoga helps a child to ride the tide of advancing puberty and thereafter to direct and channel the energy of youth.

The Physiological Importance of Yoga-asanas for Adolescents

The important physiological and physical benefits of the Yoga-asanas are that they:

* Improve circulation vital to the proper functioning of the body.

* Nourish, stimulate and maintain the vital balance of the endocrinal glands which govern growth and development.

* Help establish a regular and easy menstural cycle.

* Improve functions such as digestion and respiration so

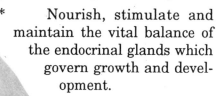

that there is more energy available for the growing child.

* Increase the supply of fresh blood to the brain thus enhancing the mental capacity.

* Strengthen the nerves whereby the endurance capacity improves.

* Promote proper structural development by working the joints.

The Psychological Importance of Yoga-asanas for Adolescents

The important psychological and emotional benefits of the Yoga-asanas are that they:

* Help a child to become self-controlled and less prone to extremes of behaviour (which tends to occur during adolescence) by regulating endocrinal functions.

* Check excessive aggression and excitability through the regulation of the adrenal glands.

* Correct brooding and melancholy in girls by regulating pituitary and pineal functions.

* Check laziness and lethargy which sometimes characterizes this phase.

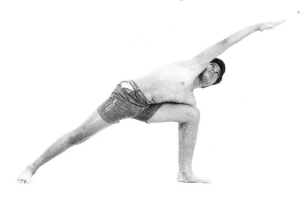

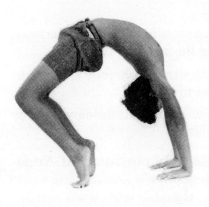

* Build up self-confidence. Remove shyness and self-consciousness.

* Control the arousal of the emerging sexual urge.

* Direct the new found energy into creative outlets.

* Create predisposition towards Yogic principles of yama and niyama so developing a child's moral-ethical character.

Notes on Yoga-asanas for Adolescents

Asanas are not merely physical movements. They have a far reaching impact on a growing child. Here are few examples:

* The Standing Poses develop the physique and build up stamina, remove stiffness and lethargy.

* The Sun Salutation Poses (the Jumpings) build up strength and stamina. They bring freshness and remove torpidity.

* The Inverted Poses sharpen the intellect. They strengthen the nerves and help regulate endocrinal functioning.

* The Cross Legged Poses and Sitting Poses create mobility in the hip, knee and ankle joints. They improve the breathing and make the mind alert.

* The Forward Bending Poses bring sobriety and calm the emotions.

* The Twisting Poses strengthen the back. They create calmness and reduce excitation.

* The Prone and the Backward Bending Poses remove dullness and provide energy.

* The Balancing Poses are challenging and expressive. On performing them a child feels a sense of achievement. They build up self-confidence.

* The Leg Movement Poses bring strength, flexibility and alignment to the joints and muscles of the legs.

* The Body Knotting Poses are challenging and demanding. They are most useful in improving the blood circulation in the vital organs.

During Menstruation:

Ideally, one should rest during menstruation for about two days. If, however, girls wish to practice Yoga-asanas during menstruation, it is quite safe to do all the asanas except for the inverted poses which should not be done on any account. Should a girl have excessive pain or bleeding or any other abnormality, the following asanas are highly recommended. Supta Vira-asana, Matsya-asana, followed by all the Forward Bending Poses, followed by Viparita Danda-asana on a chair or bench, Setu Bandha Sarvanga-asana on a bench and finally Shava-asana.

5. The Yoga Syllabus

By Geeta Iyengar

Yoga is a vast and multi-faceted subject. Teachers are perplexed as to which aspect of Yoga should be introduced in schools.

Yoga-asanas are the aspect of Yoga which should be introduced in schools. Asana is the only limb of Yoga that can be directly imparted. Properly taught and practiced, the Yoga-asanas will provide the children sound physical and mental health and lead to balanced growth. Children are basically active and outgoing by nature. They enjoy the action, movement and creativity that the asanas provide and will readily take to them. Furthermore, the asanas are safe and can easily be taught and corrected. By exposing the children to Yoga-asanas at the middle school level, interest in the subject of Yoga will be created at the right age. Later, at the college level, when these children are more mature, they can take up the higher aspects of Yoga such as pranayama, meditation and philosophy.

Which and How Many Asanas Should Children Learn

A question is often raised as to which and how many asanas should be taught in schools. Unfortunately, most schools and Yoga teachers have confined their courses to a few basic asanas when introducing Yoga as a subject i.e. Padmasana, Matsyasana, Mayurasana, Dhanurasana (also called Chakrasana), Bhujangasana, Shirsasana, Sarvangasana, Halasana and a few others.

While teaching school children one should not confine oneself to just a few asanas. Children learn quickly. Even if a child is allotted just one session of Yoga in a week he can easily learn 30 to 40 asanas in the course of a year. Obviously, if children have two or more sessions of Yoga a week, they need a syllabus with many more asanas. Children need variety and novelty. By practicing a variety of asanas children can explore a wide range of movements. The novelty is necessary to keep their interest in the subject alive. By repeating the same poses in each class, the children get bored. Though the asanas are age-old, the teacher must be innovative to keep the child's interest alive.

Progress cannot be made if the teacher insists that the child perfects one asana before introducing new asanas. While some important asanas have to be taught and repeated in each session, there are other asanas which one teaches only occasionally.

The perfection of some asanas depends on the performance of several other asanas. For example, if a group of children find it difficult to perform Padmasana, they need to practice several poses which are preparatory to Padmasana like: Gomukhasana, Virasana, Eka Pada Bhekasana, Ardha Baddha Padmottanasana, Utthitha Hasta Padangushthasana, Ardha Padmasana, etc. Similarly, to improve Halasana the cycle of Paschimottanasana-Halasana should be practiced regularly.

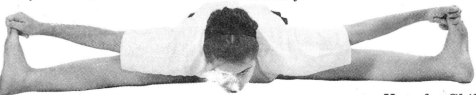

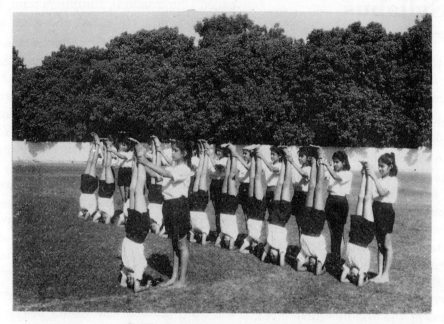

Helpful Asanas during Exams

During exams children should practice several Inverted asanas such as Shirsasana, Sarvangasana, Halasana, Setubandha Sarvangasana and Viparita Karani. These asanas stimulate and help to relieve tension. The lateral twist of the spine removes back-aches and neck pain. Shanmukhi Mudra relaxes the eyes. In fact, the Yoga syllabus for children should include asanas which remove fatigue and mental strain.

Syllabus and Guidelines

A complete and comprehensive syllabus is required to teach Yoga-asana in schools. With a rigid syllabus, however, children tend to lose interest in the class. The syllabus should begin with simple asanas and proceed towards complicated asanas. The children should first be taught the asanas which correct anatomical defects and create strength and flexibility. Having prepared the foundation properly, the teacher should proceed to teach more complicated asanas which effect the physiology and psychology of the child. Below is a general guideline which suggests the basic requirements and sequence of the Yoga course.

1. The Standing Asanas i.e. Utthitha Trikonasana
2. The Sitting Asanas i.e. Virasana
3. The Forward Bending Asanas i.e. Paschimottanasana
4. The Inverted Asanas i.e. Shirsasana
5. The Supine Asanas i.e. Matsyasana
6. The Prone Asanas i.e. Shalabhasana
7. The Lateral Twisting Asanas i.e. Bhardvajasana
8. The Backward Bending Asanas i.e. Urdhva Dhanurasana
9. The Arm Balancing Asanas i.e. Bhujapidasana

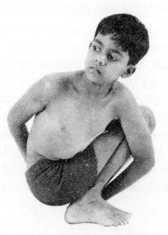

Sometimes Yoga teachers are apprehensive about teaching children a variety of asanas. For example, some teachers are afraid to teach children Upavistha Konasana, but in reality, Upavistha Konasana is quite easy for children to attempt. Unfortunately, some Yoga teachers do not practice a wide range of asanas themselves. They impose their limitations on the children and they judge the students' capabilities by their own limited capacities.

Shirsasana for Children

Some Yoga teachers are afraid to teach children Shirsasana fearing that it may strain the brain and harm the child. These fears are totally unfounded. In fact, if Shirshasana is practiced properly, it removes fatigue and rejuvenates the brain. Since children have to study a lot, they should practice Shirsasana regularly.

10. The Leg-Movement Asanas i.e. Supta Padangushthasana

11. The Body-Knotting Asanas i.e. Yoganidrasana.

Yoga-asanas are often mistaken for contortions of the body. The teacher should explain that the skilful practitioner does not contort the body. Skill in the performance of Yoga-asanas means the correct placement of the limbs, muscles and organs in the different postures.

Finally, one should note that the Yoga-asanas must be taught to children in a manner appealing to them, i.e., full of speedy and dynamic movements. If Yoga teachers fail to understand the psychology of children then "Yoga for Children" will be a big failure (See "The Dynamic Approach for Children").

On Teaching Yoga Theory

The theoretical aspects of Yoga can be introduced at the high school level but a separate theory class should not be allotted. Children do not enjoy formal classes on Yoga theory. If, on the other hand, the teacher mentions the importance of Yoga-asanas while teaching the asanas, the child will be attentive. Anatomy and physiology and many other aspects can be taught in this casual manner. Children also love listening to the meanings and the mythological stories underlying the names of asanas.

Occasionally short talks can be given on topics such as: What is Yoga, Ashtanga Yoga, Bahiranga Sadhana, morality. These talks will add to their knowledge (See Chapter "Yoga Theory for Children").

The teacher must not attempt to teach erudite concepts of *Patanjali Yoga Sutras* such as kriya Yoga, samapatti and samadhi. This sort of abstract theory is not appropriate for children as they can't relate such concepts to their day to day lives and personal experiences. The teacher must use simple explanations and information.

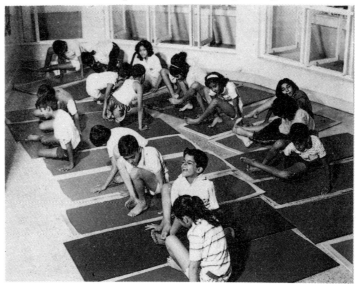

6. The Dynamic Approach for Children

By Geeta Iyengar

If children are taught too many static asanas, where they have to hold the pose and make thoughtful adjustments, they will get bored and distracted. Children need activity and enjoy motion. Children, therefore, must be taught asanas primarily in a dynamic way involving many speedy, forceful and energetic movements.

Dynamic movements activate unused joints and muscles. Stiff bodies are thereby made supple, preparing children for asanas that they could not previously do easily. New movements are achieved. The dynamic and speedy movements also have a positive effect on the mind. They destroy lethargy and remove fear complexes that hinder free movements. They instill courage in the children and perform a literal 'brain washing' which makes the children feel fresh.

To achieve a dynamic effect asanas should be combined together and performed in quick succession. Initially, the emphasis must be on speed while performing these asanas, but later speed must be combined with accuracy and grace. Here are a few examples of how asanas can be combined or strung together:

a) Perform the Surya Namaskar Cycle (also called the Jumping Poses). These include Tadasana, Urdhva Hastasana, Uttanasana, Adho Mukha Shvanasana, Urdhva Mukha Shvanasana, Chaturanga Dandasana and reverse back in a similar manner. These six poses can be practiced in various permutations and combinations.

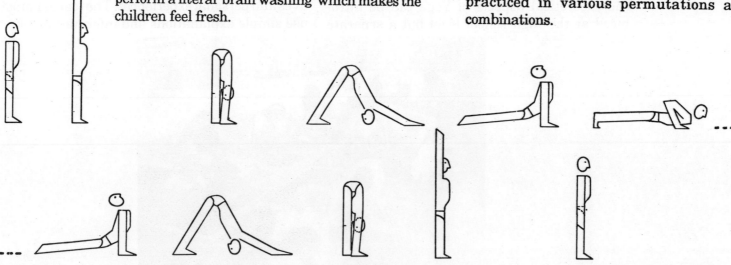

b) Perform all the Standing Poses at a stretch without returning to Tadasana each time.

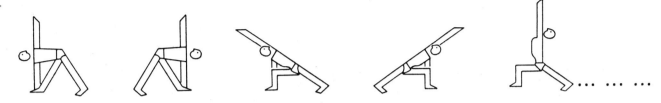

c) Practice all the Standing Poses continuously on the right side and finish with Tadasana. Then perform the Standing Poses continuously on the left side.

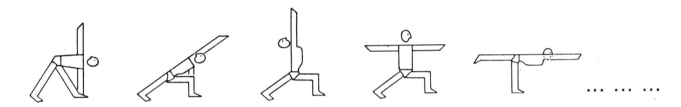

d) Blend the asanas: Utthitha Trikonasana, Ardha Chandrasana, Virabhadrasana II, Parivritta Parshvakonasana, Parivritta Trikonasana, Parshvottanasana, Urdhva Prasarita Eka Padasana, Uttitha Hasta Padangusthasana. Do these on the right side at a stretch without giving a break. The same cycle can be repeated on the left side. This can, again, have several permutations and combinations.

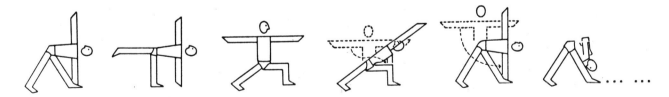

e) Combine two or more asanas and practice the sequence repeatedly e.g. Parshvottanasana Urdhva Prasarita Eka Padasana.

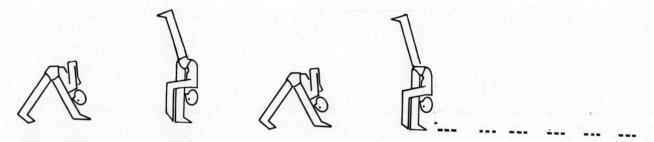

f) Do cycles blending Navasana, Halasana and each Forward Bend.

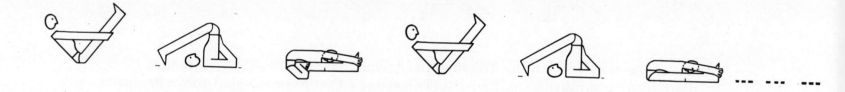

g) Combine different movements from the Surya Namaskar cycle with the Standing and the Forward Bending Poses.

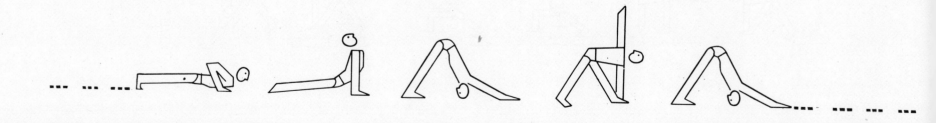

h) Do all the Forward Bending Poses continuously on the right side and then continuously on the left side.

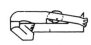 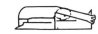 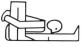 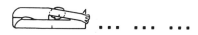

i) Combine each of the Forward Bending Poses with the Lateral Twisting Poses.

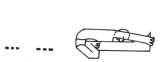   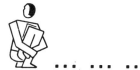

j) Combine each Forward Bending Poses with a Backward Bending Pose like Urdhva Dhanurasana or Ushtrasana.

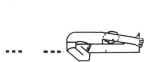 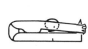   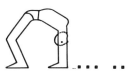

k) Form a chain of one Forward Bending asana and one Backward Bending asana.

 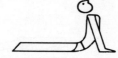  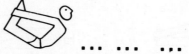 ... ...

If the students are taught in this manner they develop grace, skill, freedom, courage, quickness, steadiness, a sense of balance, agility, suppleness, sharpness and physical and mental control. The teacher can and should add several different permutations and combinations to the above mentioned examples. Thereby the children will enjoy the variety and change and derive many benefits at the same time.

7. Pranayama, Shatkriyas and Bandhas are Not for Children

By Geeta Iyengar

Having considered what should be included in the Yoga syllabus for children, let us now consider which aspects of Yoga should be omitted.

Pranayama - Controlled and Volitional Breathing

One must caution Yoga teachers against teaching children pranayama as it is not suited to the nature of children. Pranayama demands steadiness, seriousness and keen observation, whereas children are playful, naughty and restless by nature. The mass psychology of children is such that when they are together they can't easily be serious nor can they be easily controlled. If they are asked to keep their eyes closed for too long they burst out laughing. Also if the instructor points out some anatomical detail the children laugh and become mischievous. Children physically can't cope with pranayama. If children are asked to sit quietly they drop the spine (though while practicing asanas they can activate the spine better than adults). Furthermore, if children are asked to breathe consciously, they move the chest and abdomen dynamically and mechanically.

On the mental plane, pranayama is a monotonous and unexciting job for children and does not provide any outlet for their creativity. They don't find anything expressive or impressive in it, nor do they find any immediate results or any sense of achievement in the practice of pranayama.

Physiologically, pranayama is inappropriate for children. Bhastrika pranayama is dangerous for children as they can definitely damage the delicate blood vessels and brain cells. In fact, pranayama may cause children to grow old prematurely. Therefore, children should not be taught pranayama.

How then should one prepare children for the practice of pranayama which is important later in life? If, while teaching asanas, older children are made aware of their breathing pattern, that is sufficient preparation for children. See below.

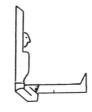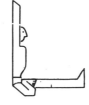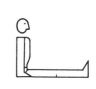

1. Normal   2. Inhale   3. Exhale   4. Inhale   5. Exhale and then normal

When the children get tired performing dynamic asanas, they can be taught to rest with the chest raised up and well opened. They will recover quickly thereby learning the importance of correct breathing through practical experience. Since asanas cleanse the inner body, certain asanas can also be used to prepare the children for pranayama without touching on the pranayamic process directly.

If, however, a teacher or parent is very keen to teach children pranayama, then Stage I of viloma pranayama (interrupted inhalation) can be taught to them for four to five minutes.

Shatikriyas - The Six Cleansing Practices

The *Hatha Yoga Pradipika* clearly states that the shatkriyas are not meant for everyone.

These kriyas are only for those whose humours are completely vitiated, for the diseased people. These kriyas are habit forming; people who habitually practice them will have trouble with routine functions such as emptying the bowels when not performing the kriyas.

The Science of Ayurveda also does not recommend the shatkriyas for children.

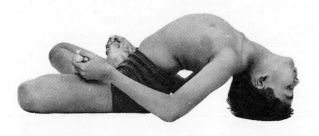

According to Ayurveda, because children under the age of fourteen years are of kapha prakriti, they should avoid all shodhana kriyas (purifying treatments) like the shatkriyas. Instead , children should be treated by shamana kriyas (pacifying treatments).

Furthermore, the shatkriyas are impractical and there is the problem of hygiene such as the availability of clean thread, clean water and other facilities required for the kriyas. In fact, saucha (cleanliness), the first of the niyamas prescribed by Patanjali, is sufficient for children. Teaching children to brush their teeth, clean their tongue, blow their nostrils lightly, move their bowels regularly, bathe and cultivate good habits is enough for them. In addition, if children regularly practice Yoga-asanas their physiological functions like digestion and excretion will greatly improve.

Bandhas - Postures Which Affect Specific Contractions

Children should not be taught uddiyana and other bandhas because by practicing these, children become excessively conscious of their lower abdomen and reproductive organs. In young children these organs are functionally dormant. If children practice these bandhas their physiology will start functioning before puberty. As a result, premature seminal discharge may occur in boys. It would be damaging to the children's health to make their physiology mature while they are still mentally immature. Thus, children should not be taught the bandhas.

8. More Asanas for Children

Because novelty and variety are the keys for teaching Yoga-asanas to children, we have described 40 more asanas here. If these asanas alongwith the 75 asanas presented in the earlier part of this book are taught to children in different permutations and combinations and with varying areas of emphasis, children will remain absorbed by the subject of Yoga for years.

Many of the asanas explained here are variations of the asanas already described in the earlier part of this book. Some asanas are new and difficult.

Asanas marked with one asterisk may be integrated into Course I of the practice sequences, those marked with two asterisks into Course II and those marked with three asterisks into Course III.

THE STANDING POSES

1. Prasarita Pada-uttana-asana II ***
(Spread-Leg Intense-Stretch Pose)
10 to 20 counts

Stand in Tada-asana. Fold your palms behind your back. Keeping your palms in this position do Prasarita Pada-uttana-asana I.

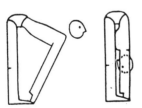

2. Pada-angustha-asana **
(Big Toe Pose)
10 to 20 counts

(i) A preparation to Uttana-asana. Stand in Tada-asana. Bend forward. Hook your big toes with your thumb, index and middle fingers. Keep your knees and arms straight and dip your back in. Look up. Pause

(ii) Then bend your elbows and bring your head to your knees.

3. Ardha Baddha Padma Uttana-asana ***
(Half-Restrained-Lotus Intense-Stretch Pose)
(15 to 20 counts each side)

Stand in Tada-asana. Bend your right leg as in Padma-asana. Swing your right arm behind your back and catch hold of your right foot. Bend forward as in Uttana-asana. Pause. Then do the pose on the other side.

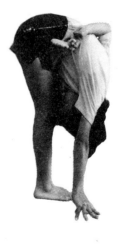

THE SITTING AND THE CROSS-LEGGED POSES

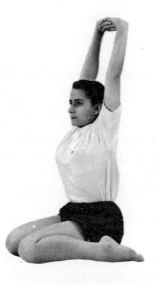

4. Vira-asana III *
(Warrior Pose III)
10 to 20 counts

Sit in Vira-asana. Interlock your fingers and raise your arms as in Parvata-asana. Pause. Then bring the arms down, change the interlock of the fingers and repeat the pose.

5. Swastika-asana *
(Swastika, the Good-Luck Symbol Pose)
30 to 60 counts

This is a simple cross-legged position. Start from Danda-asana. Then bend your right leg and tuck your right foot under your left thigh. Then bend your left leg and rest the left foot on the right thigh. Sit very erect. Position the hands in Jnana Mudra.

6. Simha-asana *
(Lion Pose I)
10 counts

This is a simple variation of Simha-asana for those who cannot cross their legs in Padma-asana.

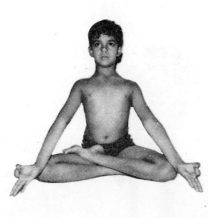

Position your legs as in Lola-asana. Rest your palms on your knees and spread your fingers. Then stick out your tongue, look at the tip of your nose and breathe through the mouth. After a few breaths change the crossing of your legs and repeat the pose.

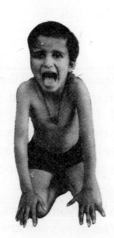

7. Yoga Mudra-asana *
(Yogic Seal Pose)
15 counts

This is a simple version of Yoga Mudra-asana. Sit in Padma-asana. Take your hands behind your back. Interlock your fingers. Then bend forward raising your arms to a perpendicular position behind your back. Pause. Then bring your arms down, interlock your fingers the other way, change the crossing of your legs and repeat the pose.

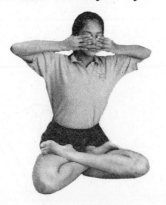

8. Shanmukhi Mudra ***
(Lord Kartikeya Mudra)
30 to 60 counts

Sit in Padma-asana with your eyes closed. Plug your ears with your thumbs. Then cover your eyes with your index and middle fingers. Next place your ring fingers on your nostrils and partially block your nasal passages. Lastly, rest your small fingers on your upper lip. Keep your elbows lifted and level with your shoulders. Be steady and stay a while in this position.

THE INVERTED POSES

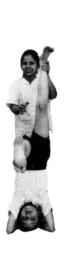

9. Shirsha-asana II **
(Head Stand)
1 to 3 minutes

(i) Kneel in front of a folded blanket. Place the crown of the head on the blanket and the palms on the floor forming a tripod.

(ii) Raise your knees off the floor and walk towards your head.

(iii) Raise your legs upwards, together or one at a time.

(iv) Come into an inverted position and balance. Lift up and broaden your shoulders. Do not widen your elbows. Stay a while, then come down.

10. Prasarita Pada Shirsha-asana ***
(Spread-Leg Head-Stand)
10 to 15 counts

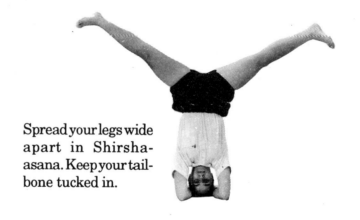

Spread your legs wide apart in Shirsha-asana. Keep your tail-bone tucked in.

Children may help each other in Shirsha-asana. Here is a technique:

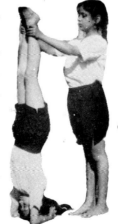

a. Always stand behind your partner.

b. After your partner has positioned the arms and head ask your partner to raise one leg up.

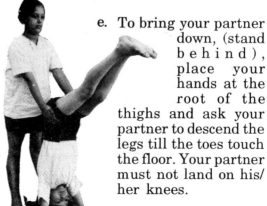

c. Grab hold of the leg (from behind) and pull it up to a perpendicular position. The other leg will come up by itself.

d. Support your partner and ensure that she/he is straight. Let go occasionally so that she/he learns to balance.

e. To bring your partner down, (stand behind), place your hands at the root of the thighs and ask your partner to descend the legs till the toes touch the floor. Your partner must not land on his/her knees.

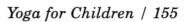

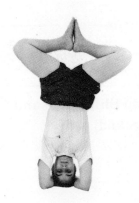

11. Baddha Kona-asana in Shirsha-asana ***
(Restrained Angle Pose in Head-Stand)
10 to 15 counts

Perform Shirsha-asana. Then bend your legs as in Baddha Kona-asana. Press the soles of your feet together and move your knees back.

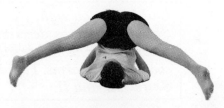

12. Eka Pada Shirsha-asana ***
(One Leg Head-Stand)
10 counts each side

Perform Shirsha-asana. Then, keeping your left leg upright bring your right leg half-way down or all the way to the floor. Keep both knees straight. Pause. Then do the pose on the other side.

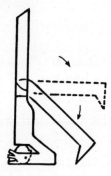

14. Supta Kona-asana *
(Lying Angle Pose)
15 to 20 counts

Perform Hala-asana. Then spread your legs wide apart. Keep your back erect and knees straight.

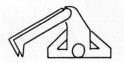

13. Urdhva Padma-asana in Shirsha-asana ***
(Raised Lotus Pose in Head-Stand)
10 to 20 counts

Perform Shirsha-asana. Then cross your legs as in Padma-asana. Tuck your tail-bone in and move your knees back. Pause. Then change the crossing of your legs and repeat the pose.

15. Parshva Hala-asana **
(Sideways Plough Pose)
10 to 20 counts each side

Perform Hala-asana. Move both legs to your right side till the feet are in line with your right shoulder. Keep the back erect and the buttocks level. Straighten your knees. Pause. Then take your legs to the left side.

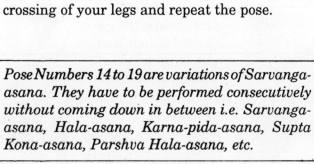

Pose Numbers 14 to 19 are variations of Sarvanga-asana. They have to be performed consecutively without coming down in between i.e. Sarvanga-asana, Hala-asana, Karna-pida-asana, Supta Kona-asana, Parshva Hala-asana, etc.

16. Eka Pada Sarvanga-asana **
(One-Leg Sarvanga-asana)
10 to 20 counts each side

Perform Sarvanga-asana. Keeping the left leg upright, bring your right leg half-way down or to the floor. Don't bend your knees or tilt your body. Pause. Then repeat the pose on the other side.

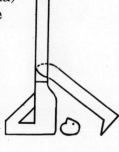

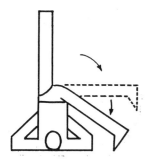

17. Parshva Eka Pada Sarvanga-asana **
(Sideways One-Leg Sarvanga-asana)
10 to 20 counts each side

Perform Sarvanga-asana. Turn your right foot sideways. Then descend your right leg sideways down towards the floor. Keep your left leg perpendicular. Don't tilt the body or bend the knees. Pause. Then repeat the pose on the other side.

18. Urdhva Padma-asana in Sarvanga-asana ***
(Raised Lotus-Pose in Sarvanga-asana)
15 to 20 counts each side

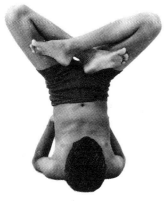

Perform Sarvanga-asana. Then cross your legs as in Padma-asana. Keep your back erect and tuck in your tail-bone. Pause. Then do the pose crossing your legs the other way.

19. Pinda-asana in Sarvanga-asana ***
(Embryo Pose in Sarvanga-asana)
10 to 20 counts

Perform Urdhva Padma-asana in Sarvanga-asana. Then bring your crossed legs towards your head. Pause. Then return to Sarvanga-asana, change the crossing of the legs and repeat the pose.

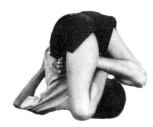

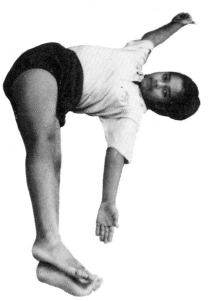

20. Pincha Mayura-asana ***
(Feathered Peacock Pose)
10 to 30 counts

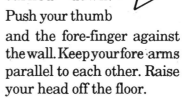

(i) Kneel facing a wall. Rest your forearms on the floor with palms turned down. Push your thumb and the fore-finger against the wall. Keep your fore arms parallel to each other. Raise your head off the floor.

(ii) Raise your knees up. Then kick your legs upwards one at a time.

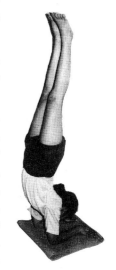

(iii) Come into an inverted position and rest your heels against the wall. Curve your neck back and raise your head and shoulders up. Be careful that your palms don't join and that your elbows don't spread out. Stay a while in the pose and then come down.

THE SUPINE POSES

21. Jathara Parivartana-asana ***
(Stomach Turning Pose)
5 counts each side

(i) Raise your legs to 90° as in Urdhva Prasarita Pada-asana. Stretch your arms sideways with the palms turned up.

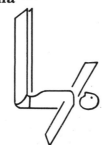

(ii) Slowly take both legs towards your right palm. Pause when your feet are just six inches off the floor. Keep your knees straight.

(iii) Bring your legs back to 90° then do the pose on the left side. Finally, return to Urdhva Prasarita Pada-asana and then descend the legs to floor.

22. Paryanka-asana ***

(Couch Pose)

5 to 10 counts

Lie in Supta Vira-asana. Place your palms under your shoulders, arch your back and rest the crown of your head on the floor. Then cross your arms overhead.

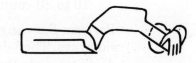

THE FORWARD BENDING POSES

23. Kroncha-asana ***

(Heron Pose)

10 to 20 counts each side

Sit as in Trianga Mukha Eka Pada Paschima-uttana-asana with the left leg extended and the right leg bent as in Vira-asana. Then slightly bend your left knee and clasp the left foot with both hands. Now raise your left leg upwards. Keeping the left knee poker stiff, bring the left leg to your head. Pause. Then do the pose on the other side.

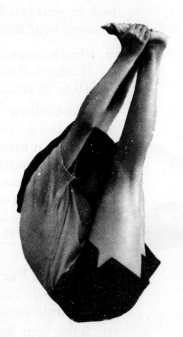

24. Urdhva Mukha Paschima-uttana-asana ***

(Upwards-Face Paschima-uttana-asana)

10 to 15 counts

Sit in Danda-asana. Bend your knees and clasp your feet with both hands. Raise your legs upwards. Keeping your legs poker stiff, bring your knees to your head. Balance.

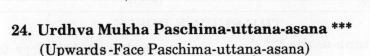

THE TWISTING POSE

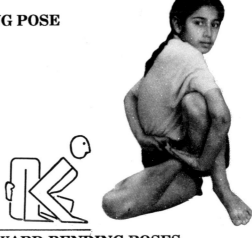

25. Marichi-asana IV ***

(Sage Marichi Pose)

10 to 15 counts

(i) Sit as in Marichi-asana II with your left leg in Padma-asana and the right leg bent upwards.

(ii) Wrap your left arm around your right knee and then clasp hands behind your back. Pause. Then repeat the pose on the other side.

THE PRONE AND THE BACKWARD BENDING POSES

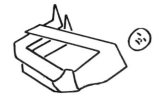

26. Parshva Dhanur-asana **

(Sideways Bow Pose)
Repeat a few times

Perform Dhanur-asana. Then roll over onto your right side. Come back to Dhanur-asana and then roll onto your left side. You may also rock back and forth.

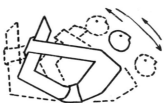

> *Backward-Bending poses such as Urdhva Dhanur-asana, Viparita-Danda-asana and Kapota-asana can be done with greater ease if children first prepare themselves by bending back-wards on chairs (as described in the Chapter on "props").*

27. Urdhva Dhanur-asana II ***

(Raised Bow Pose)
Repeat a few times

(i) Stand in Tada-asana with the feet six to nine inches apart. Keep your feet parallel to each other.

(ii) Rest your hands on your hips and curve back keeping your knees straight.

(iii) Then take your arms overhead. Bend your knees and curve further. Keep your eyes on your finger tips. (Use a wall to learn)

(iv) Drop your hands on the floor. Pause.

(v) Then come up with a swing or bend your elbows and gently descend to the floor.

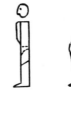

 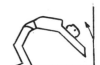

Urdhva Dhanur-asana I and Urdhva Dhanur-asana II can be made more enjoyable and challenging by asking the child to do the following:

- *Move your feet closer to your hands*
- *Move your hands closer to your feet*
- *Join your feet and knees*
- *Raise your heels, lift your spine as high as possible and then gently descend your heels without dropping the height of your spine.*
- *Begin the pose with your wrists touching the wall. Raise up your body. Then move your feet closer to your hands and press your chest against the wall (without bending your elbows)*
- *Place your hand on a ledge or brick and then do the pose (See Chapter on props)*
- *Do the pose with your feet on a height, i.e. a ledge or a brick*

28. Eka Pada Urdhva Dhanur-asana ***
(One Leg Inverted Bow Pose)
5 to 10 counts each side

Perform Urdhva Dhanur-asana. Then raise your right leg high up in the air, keeping the knee straight. Pause. Descend the right leg and then raise your left leg up.

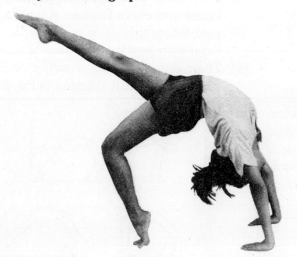

29. Viparita Danda-asana ***
(Inverted Rod Pose)
30 to 60 counts

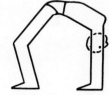

(i) Perform Urdhva Dhanur-asana.

(ii) Bend your elbows and rest the crown of your head on the floor. Interlock your fingers behind your head (as for Shirsha-asana). Rest your elbows on the floor keeping your forearms in contact with your ears as in Shirsha-asana.

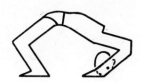

(iii) Move your feet away from your head. Straighten your knees if you can and join your feet. Keep your chest well opened and the tailbone lifted. Pause a while in this pose.

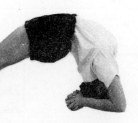

(iv) Then bend your knees, place your palms on the floor and gradually come down.

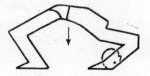

THE ARM BALANCING POSES

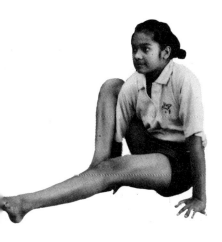

30. Eka Hasta Bhuja-asana ***
(One Arm Bhuja-asana)
10 counts each side

Stand in Uttana-asana. Then bend down and place your right leg over your right upper arm as in Bhuja-pida-asana. Insert your left leg between your arms and extend it forward, keeping it in the air. Balance for a while, then do the pose on other side.

31. Dwi Hasta Bhuja-asana ***
(Two Arms Bhuja-asana)
10 counts

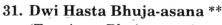

Stand as in Uttana-asana. Place both legs over the upper arm as in Bhuja-pida-asana. Balance for a while without crossing the ankles.

32. Tittibha-asana ***
(Firefly Pose)
10 counts

Perform Dwi Hasta Bhuja-asana. Then straigthen your knees and stretch out your legs.

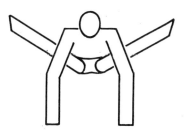

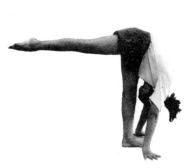

33. Mayura-asana ***
(Peacock Pose)
10 counts

(i)   Kneel. Place your palms on the floor fingers pointing towards your knees.

(ii) Bend your elbows. Then lean forward and rest your stomach on the elbows. Keep your head raised off the floor.

(iii) Straighten your legs and raise them off the floor.

      Balance keeping your body parallel to the floor.

34. Purva-uttana-asana **
(Eastern Stretch Pose)
10 to 15 counts

(i)   Sit in Danda-asana. Place your palms on the floor behind you.

(ii) Raise your hips and thighs off the floor taking all the body weight on your hands and feet. Contract the buttocks and throw your head back.

THE LEG MOVEMENT POSES

35. Urdhva Prasarita Eka Pada-asana ***
(Upwards Stretched One Leg Pose)
10 to 15 counts each side

Perform Uttana-asana. Then raise your left leg high up in the air. Keep both knees poker stiff. Pause. Then do the pose on the other side.

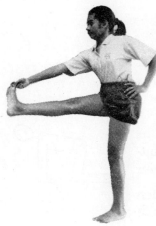

36. Utthitha Hasta Pada-angustha-asana ***
(Extended Arm Leg Big Toe Pose)
10 counts on each side

Stand in Tada-asana with the hands on the hips. Bend your right leg and hook your big toe with your right thumb, index and middle fingers. Then extend the right leg and the right arm forward. Keep both knees absolutely straight. Pause. Then do the pose on the other side.

37. Supta Pada-angustha-asana ***
(Lying Down Leg Big Toe Pose)
10 counts each side

(i) Lie flat on your back with the legs stretched out and the knees straight. Rest your left hand on your left thigh.

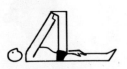

(ii) Raise the right leg and hook the right big toe with your right thumb, index and middle fingers. Straighten your leg and pause a while.

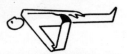

(iii) Now take the right leg sideways down towards the floor without bending the knee. Do not disturb the left leg.

(iv) Repeat the movements on the left side.

THE BODY-KNOTTING POSES

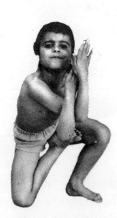

38. Vatayana-asana ***
(Horse Pose)
10 counts each side

(i) Stand in Tada-asana. Place your left leg as in Padma-asana. Then bend and rest your left knee on the floor.

(ii) Entwine your arms as in Garuda-asana. Pause. Then repeat the pose on the other side.

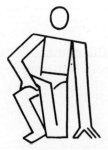

39. Eka Pada Shirsha-asana ***
(One Leg Head Pose) 10 counts each side

(i) Sit as in Janu Shirsha-asana with your left leg extended and the right leg bent. Then lift up the right leg, pull it behind the right shoulder and rest the right foot behind the neck.

(ii) Try to sit erect. Fold your palms in front of your chest. Pause. Then do the pose on the other side.

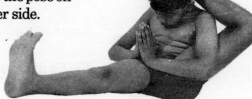

40. Yoga Nidra-asana ***

(Sleep of the Yogi Pose. The back is the bed, the feet are the pillow and the arms are the blanket)
10 to 20 counts

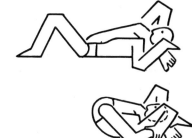

(i) Lie on your back. Then take the right leg behind your shoulder as in Eka Pada Shirsha-asana.

(ii) Then also take your left leg behind your shoulder. Cross the ankles behind the neck.

(iii) Then take your arms around your back and clasp hands. Pause, then change the crossing of the ankles and repeat the pose.

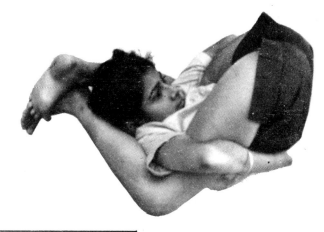

Shava-asana

During Shava-asana children are often restless and fidgety. To keep them quiet and attentive, the teacher may tell them stories (which reinforce the values of yama and niyama).

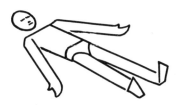

9. Yoga Props for Children

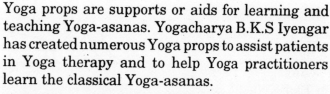

Yoga props are supports or aids for learning and teaching Yoga-asanas. Yogacharya B.K.S Iyengar has created numerous Yoga props to assist patients in Yoga therapy and to help Yoga practitioners learn the classical Yoga-asanas.

In this chapter we have, confined ourselves to using only simple objects from everyday life when describing how Yoga props can be used by children. These will help a child develop strength and flexibility and provide variety in a child's Yoga practice.

The Floor: A line on the floor can be a useful learning and teaching aid. Teach children to stand on a line and align their bodies viz-a-viz the lines while practicing asanas, particularly the Standing Poses. This teaches them the basis of *alignment* in Yoga-asanas.

The Wall: Walls can serve as useful props. They provide invaluable support when a child begins learning Inverted Poses like Shirsha-asana and Adho Mukha Vriksha-asana.

Learning Shirsha-asana Against A Wall.

1. Place your blanket against a wall preferably in a corner or against an edge where two walls meet.
2. Rest your forearms on the blanket and interlock your fingers. The knuckles must touch the wall.
3. Come into an inverted position. Be sure that you are not tilted to a side.
4. Only the heels should rest against the wall. Broaden and lift your shoulders. Tighten the buttock muscles. Stay a while.

Difficult arm - balancing poses like Baka-asana can also be learned with the help of a wall, resting the toes against a wall.

Children can gain confidence and flexibility by practicing Urdhva Dhanur-asana using the wall for support. (See page 159)

The wall can also provide resistance whereby the pupils can improve their pose as in Adho Mukha Shava-asana.(Place fingers against a wall)

Wall Ropes: (Traditionally called Yoga Kurunta) A wide range of movements can be performed on wall ropes. These movements create flexion and extension and are very good for developing a growing child's muscles and promoting growth. Besides strengthening the back and making the

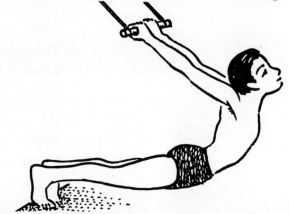

spine supple, they also enable the children to perform difficult poses. One could loop ropes around step ladders in a gymnasium or hooks on a wall.

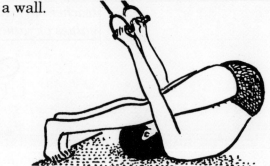

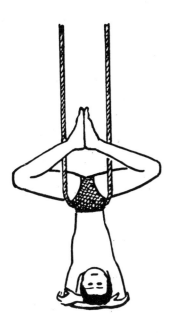

The Ceiling Ropes: Ropes can also be suspended from rafters or from hooks in the ceiling

Children love to hang upside down in 'Rope Shirsha-asana' from these ceiling ropes. This stress-free version of Shirsha-asana is beneficial for all children because the brain and the pineal and pituitary glands are supplied with fresh blood in this position. Even a beginner can stay comfortably in this inverted position.

The Chair: Sarvanga- asana can be done with the help of chair. Here is the method:

1. Place a bolster or two folded blankets near the front legs of a chair. Then sit side-ways on the chair.
2. Swing your legs onto the back rest of the chair and hold the sides of the back-rest.
3. Gradually lean back till your shoulders rest on the bolster or blankets and rest the back of your head on the floor.
4. Extend your arms backwards within the legs of the chair and hold the back legs of the chair, if possible.

It is easy for a child to stay a while in Sarvanga-asana performed in this manner. This pose is very effective in removing fatigue and refreshing the child. The inversion leads to healthy blood circulation in the thyroid gland and the brain.

Chairs can also provide useful support to prepare the back for Backward-Bending Poses. Here is the method to perform Viparita Danda-asana on the chair.

1. Insert your legs in the gap between the back rest and the seat of a chair:
2. Hold the back rest, bend your knees and gradually lie back.
3. Insert your arms between the legs of the chair (under the seat) and hold the back legs if possible. Straighten your knees and press your toes and heels to the wall. Look at the floor. Stay up to five minutes in this pose.
4. To come up, hold the back rest of the chair, bend your knees and come up with a swing.

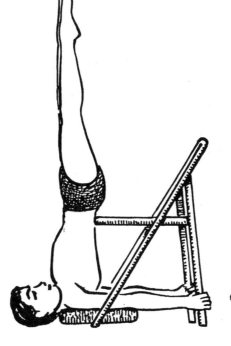

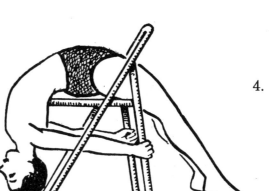

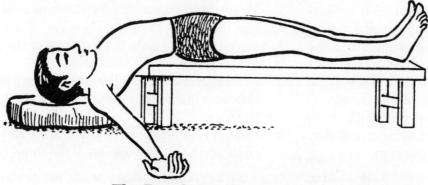

Often stiff or heavy children are not able to raise themselves off the floor in Urdhva Dhanur-asana. Resting their hands on bricks placed against a wall,   (or on a ledge about five inches high) will enable them to lift up more easily.

The Bench: Benches can be put to good use to support children in Setu Bandha Sarvanga-asana. This resting pose performs wonders to calm the nerves, rest the brain and refresh the child. This pose can be done by girls during menstruation.

Since children find Forward Bending Poses difficult and unappealing, the teacher can make these poses more endurable for children by asking a child to sit on a bench, the heels on the floor, and then to bend forward.

A bench can also serve as a support to perform Half Hala-asana: rest the toes on a bench.

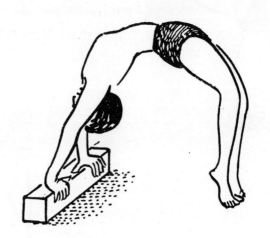

The Brick: Stiff children can't do Ardha Chandra-asana easily as their palms don't reach the floor. They tend to get disheartened with such poses. A vertical brick gives them the support they require to learn the pose. Over time the brick can be placed horizontally and when they advance in their practice they can dispense with it.

A brick provides useful resistance between the palms when older children learn to perform Pincha Mayura-asana.

The Belt: Most children find it difficult to keep their elbows parallel to each other in Sarvanga-asana. They tend to spread their elbows too far apart. This leads to a faulty pose where the tail-bone projects back and the legs come forward. A belt can be used effectively to keep the elbows in place and so correct this defect.

Some children find it difficult to stay a while in Padma-asana or to perform variations like Matsya-asana. A belt can be used to bind the knees so that children can learn to perform these poses properly.

Pillows and Bolsters: Pillows and bolsters are especially useful when a child is suffering from some ailment or injury. They can be used to give support to the unwell child in several ways, to provide relief and help in recuperation.

Blankets: Beginners have trouble staying in Sarvanga-asana for a few minutes. They can be taught to do this in the following manner:

1. Place two or three neatly folded blankets one a top the other on the floor.

2. Lie on your back with your shoulders resting on the blankets, the neck on the edge and the back of the head on the floor.

3. Then perform Sarvanga-asana.

When Sarvanga-asana is done in this manner children can lift the spine up, open the chest and stay a while in the pose. This is particularly useful for fat children.

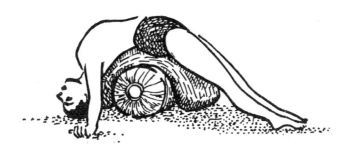

10. Yoga Theory for Children

This chapter contains a selection of theoretical and philosophical topics which will enrich a child's understanding of Yoga. The most effective manner of presenting this matter to children would be to talk informally and spontaneously during the course of the regular asana classes. The teacher should use plenty of stories, examples and anecdotes and the subject should be made relevant to the lives of children. Only the simplest aspects of theory ought to be presented to the little children, for example moral stories on yama, niyama, prayers and about the origin of asana.

WHAT IS YOGA?

The word Yoga means to join, unite or merge. It is derived from the sanskrit root *yuj*. Yoga is a science and an art. The practice of Yoga integrates the body with the mind and the mind with the soul, thereby helping us to understand our own natures and to live harmoniously with our fellow men.

Yoga can be practiced by all irrespective of race, colour, caste, creed, sex and age.

Most people are aware of only two aspects of Yoga, the asanas and meditation. Yoga is more than these two aspects. It is, in fact, an eight-fold path called Ashtanga Yoga.

ASHTANGA YOGA-The Eight Fold Path

Ashtanga Yoga or the eight limbs of Yoga are:

i) **Yama** The universal commandments. These are:

Ahimsa	-	Non-violence
Satya	-	Truth and honesty
Asteya	-	Non-covetousness
Brahmacharya	-	Continence and self-control
Aparigraha	-	Non-accumulation of needless wealth

ii) **Niyama** - The personal disciplines. These are:

Saucha	-	Cleanliness and purity
Santosha	-	Satisfaction and contentment
Tapas	-	Austerity, ability to bear hardship
Svadhyaya	-	Introspection
Ishvara Pranidhana	-	Faith in God

iii) **Asana** - Postures

iv) **Pranayama** - Control of breath and bio-energy

v) **Pratyahara** - Withdrawal of the sense organs from the objects of sense

vi) **Dharana** - Intense concentration for developing inner vision

vii) **Dhyana** - Meditation, uninterrupted and deep concentration for a prolonged period

viii) **Samadhi** - The goal of Yoga, attained after a prolonged period of dhyana. Just as a river merges into the ocean and becomes one with it, so also the individual self merges into the Universal Spirit and becomes one. Peace and happiness are experienced as all polarities such as pain and pleasure, good and bad vanish.

Only the first three limbs of Ashtanga Yoga, yama, niyama and asana are relevant for children.

SADHANA - The Quest

Sadhana implies a quest or study. There are three kinds of sadhanas.

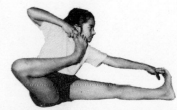

Bahiranga Sadhana (bahir-outer, anga - body) is the quest for external purity. Bahiranga sadhana consists of following the moral and ethical principles of yama and niyama for character building, and the practice of asanas for cleansing and maintaining the health of the body.

Antaranga Sadhana (antar-inner, anga - body) is the quest for inner purity. In antaranga sadhana the practitioner strives to cleanse and control his mind and his senses through the practice of pranayama and pratyahara.

Antaratma Sadhana (antar - inner, atma - soul, self) is the quest of the soul. Here the aspirant penetrates into the innermost aspects of his being through the practice of dharana, dhyana and samadhi.

Only bahiranga sadhana is for children.

PRAYERS

Prayers are a part of bahiranga sadhana. Children enjoy praying, especially praying aloud. Children are essentially pious by nature, free from doubts and biases.

Prayers inspire a child towards betterment. They help mould a character which is respectful, reviential and devout. Repetition of prayers before Yoga classes helps "set the mood". Children immediately calm down.

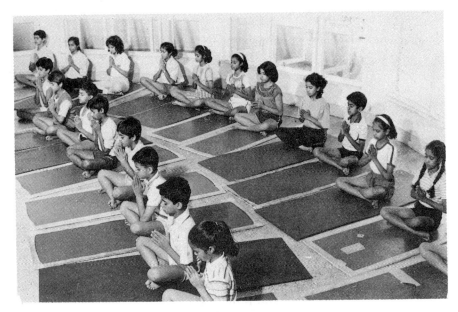

A few sanskrit prayers are given below. These can be repeated before and after the Yoga classes. These prayers are dedicated to Sage Patanjali, the founder of Yoga, to one's Guru and to the great Gods who create, sustain and dissolve the world (teachers may instead use prayers from their own tradition).

Yogena cittasya padena vacham
Malam sharirasya ca vaidyakena
Yopa' karot tam pravaram muninam
Patanjalim pranjalir anato' smi
Abahu-purushakaram
Shankha - chakarsi-dharinam
Sahashra-shirsam shvetam
Pranamami Patanjalim

To the noblest of sages, Patanjali,
Who gave Yoga for serenity of mind,
Grammer for purity of speech,
And Medicine for perfection of the body, I bow:
I prostrate before Patanjali,
Whose upper body has a human form,
Whose hands hold a conch and disc,
Who is crowned by a thousand-headed cobra,
O incarnation of Adisesa, my salutation to Thee.

Gurur-Brahama Gurur-Vishnu
Gurur-Devo Mahesvarah.
Gurur Sakshat Paru -Brahma
Tasmai Sri-Guruve Namah.

The Guru is verily Brahma, verily Vishnu
and verily Shiva too.
The Guru is in fact the Brahman (the Universal Being)
therefore I humbly bow to him.

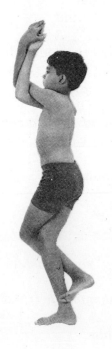

ANATOMY AND PHYSIOLOGY

Regular practice of the asanas ignites a child's curiosity about human anatomy and physiology. Likewise, knowledge about anatomy and physiology renders the study of asanas extremely interesting. During the course of a regular asana class the teacher can easily point out and name the important bones and muscles of the body.

Children learn subjectively about their bodies by practicing the Yoga asanas because every part of the body comes into play while performing these varied movements. During the course of an asana class the teacher should also indicate how the asanas work and benefit different parts of the child's body.

NAMES OF ASANAS

Children like learning the names of asanas, saying them aloud and pronouncing them correctly. They wish to understand the meaning of the names of asanas and to hear the stories, myths and legends underlying these names.

Because many asanas are inspired by nature and animals, the teacher could also trace and relate these asanas to their sources. Children are fascinated by the natural world and this approach inspires them to learn and practice the asanas.

GURU-SHISYA - The Teacher and the Pupil

A sound relationship between the guru and the shisya, the master and pupil, is the foundation for progress on the path of Yoga.

Gu means darkness and *ru* means light. The Guru is therefore the spiritual teacher, the guide, the master who leads us out of the darkness of ignorance into the light of knowledge. A guru oversees the progress of his pupil in every aspect of life; physical, moral, emotional and intellectual. He guides his disciples with faith, compassion and patience.

A shisya or pupil can be of four kinds. The ancient *Shiva Samhita* text describes them as follows:

The *mrud* is the feeble student. He has bad habits and a bad character. He criticizes his teacher and others and is cowardly.

The *madhyama* is the average student. He is moderate in his ways and wishes to improve himself.

The *adhimatra* is the good student. He is noble, truthful, brave, respectful and intent on the practice of Yoga.

The *adhimatratama* is the most superior student. He is of very good character, courageous, free from fear and independent, intelligent, studious and learned in the scriptures. He is self-controlled, regular in food, clean, generous, helpful, forgiving and gentle in speech. He is firm and not moody. He is worshipful of his Guru.

PURUSHA-ARTHAS - The Aims of Life

The ancient sages observed that man has four basic instincts or aims in life, known as the purusha-arthas. These are: dharma, artha, kama and moksha.

Dharma is the urge towards right thinking and right living.

Artha is the urge to earn honestly and acquire material wealth.

Kama is the urge to experience and enjoy the pleasures of life.

Moksha is the ultimate urge or aim to renounce the world and attain spiritual liberation.

FOUR ASHRAMAS-Stages of Life

To enable man to fulfil his four basic urges and aims, the ancients prescribed a four-fold division of a man's life span. These four divisions or stages are called ashramas. Each ashrama is, theoretically, of twenty five years duration.

Brahmacharya ashrama is the first stage in a person's life, that of a celibate student. The person lives a disciplined life devoted to studies (particularly, moral and religious).

Grahastya ashrama is the second stage, that of a man as a house-holder. The man marries, begets children, works and earns in order to maintain his family.

Vanaprastha ashrama is the third stage. With his children grown-up, the man now retires from worldly affairs and active family life. He serves as a counsellor to his family, meanwhile preparing himself inwardly for total withdrawal.

Sanyasa ashrama is the final stage in a man's life wherein he renounces all worldly bonds. He devotes himself entirely to the service of God and the attainment of salvation.

FOUR MARGS - Paths to Salvation

For attaining the cherished goal of salvation, the ancients laid down four paths or margs known as Jnana, Karma, Bhakti and Yoga.

Jnana marg - The Path of knowledge. Discriminating between what is right and wrong, real and unreal.

Karma marg - The Path of Action. Serving humanity without any thought of reward.

Bhakti marg - The Path of Devotion. Developing love and oneness with God and all creation.

Yoga marg - The Path of Integration. Cleansing the body, controlling and senses and restraining the fluctuations of the mind.

SHAD DARSHANA - Six Views

Amongst Hindus there are six orthodox schools of philosphy which explain the nature of man and the universe. These six different views are known as shad darshana. All six darshanas are based on the sacred Vedic texts, they endorse rebirth and they all aim at salvation. These six darshanas are:

Nyaya - Founder Gautama. Based on logic and reason.

Vaisheshika - Founder Kanada. Stresses notions on space, time, matter, cause, etc. and is supplementary to nyaya.

Samkhya - Founder Kapila. Gives a view of creation based on 25 different elements.

Yoga - Founder Patanjali. Provides a practical and dynamic path to salvation (i.e. Ashtanga Yoga). Follows the samkhya view of creation but adds to it the belief in God.

Mimamsa - Founder Jaimini. Stresses right action and the performance of religious rituals as explained in the Vedas.

Vedanta - Founder Badarayana. Emphasizes the path of knowledge and the search for the deep truths found in the Vedas.

IMPORTANT TEXTS

The most important text for the study of Yoga is *Yoga Sutras of Patanjali*. In merely 196 aphorisms Patanjali expounds a most brilliant and profound philosophy. This text consists of four chapters called padas.

Samadhi pada – The first chapter is intended for the advanced practitioner. It deals with experiences just preceding samadhi.

Sadhana pada – Is for the novice and explains how to begin.

Vibhuti pada – Speaks of miraculous powers and cautions against them.

Kaivalya pada – Explains the state of kaivalya, the apex of Yoga.

The *Mahabharata*, *Ramayana*, relevant portions of the *Bhagavad Gita* and *Upanishads* and stories from the *Puranas* provide great inspiration to children.

HATHA YOGA AND RAJA YOGA

Hatha means force or determination. Force and determination are required to practice Hatha Yoga. In addition *ha* means sun and *tha* means moon; just as positive and negative currents produce energy, Hatha Yoga also produces energy and force.

Raja means a king.. Raja Yoga leads to mastery over one's body and mind.

The classical text on Yoga, *Hatha Yoga Pradipika* states that both Hatha Yoga and Raja Yoga lead to the same goal, liberation.

Yogacharya B.K.S. Iyengar explains, "Both are Moksha Shastras (Sciences of Freedom). They guide man to climb the ladder of spirituality. Hatha Yoga starts with the body and ends with the soul. Raja Yoga starts with the mind and climbs down the body and uplifts again. Both criss-cross other and reach the destiny of peace, poise and plenty."

YOGIC VIEW OF CREATION

Ishwara	– God
Spirit	– Purusha
Prakriti	– Matter
Mahat	– Great productive principle
Ahamkara	– Self-consciousness
Buddhi	– Intellect
Manas	– Mind
Tanmatras	– Subtle Substances: Taste, Touch, Form, Sound, Smell
Jnanaindriyas	– Organs of Perception: Eyes, Nose, Ears, Tongue, Skin
Karmaindriyas	– Organs of Action: Legs, Arms, Speech, Excretory and Reproductive Organs
Mahabhutas	– Pure Elements – Earth, Water, Fire, Air, Ether
Tri Gunas	– The Three Qualities – All matter is constituted and pervaded by three basic qualities, gunas:
Sattva	– Pure and good
Rajas	– Energetic, active and passionate
Tamas	– Dull, inert and ignorant

YOGIC VIEW OF THE BODY

Yogic texts describe the body as being made up of five interpenetrating layers or sheaths called koshas. The investigation and harmonization of these layers is the aim of Yoga.

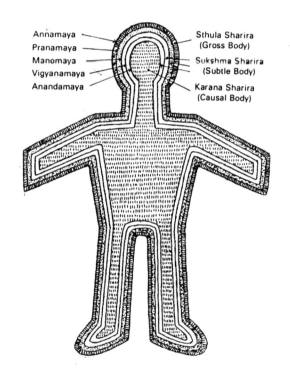

Annamaya-kosha - Anatomical sheath
Pranamaya-kosha - Physiological sheath
Manomaya-kosha - Mental sheath
Vigyanamaya-kosha - Intellectual sheath
Anandamaya-kosha - Sheath of joy (or spiritual sheath)

There is also a three-fold division of the body:

Sthula Sharira	-	Gross body (i.e. annamaya-kosha)
Sukshma Sharira	-	Subtle body (i.e. pranamaya, manomaya and vigyanamaya-kosha)
Karna Sharira	-	Causal body or innermost body (i.e. Anandamaya-kosha)

YOGIC VIEW OF THE MIND

Chitta Vrittis	-	The mind (chitta) is capable of five basic functions or modifications (vrittis). These can either cause pain or pleasure.
Pramana	-	A correct notion
Viparyaya	-	A wrong notion
Vikalpa	-	Uncertainty, fancy, imagination
Nidra	-	Sleep
Smriti	-	Memory
Kleshas	-	There are five conditions which always bring pain or misery (klesha):
Avidya	-	Ignorance
Asmita	-	Arrogance
Raga	-	Attachment
Dvesha	-	Aversion
Abhinivesha	-	Clinging to life

Different States of the Mind	- There are five different categories used to describe the mind:
Mudha	- Dull, foolish
Kshipta	- neglected, distracted
Vikshipta	- bewildered, agitated
Ekagra	- Attentive
Niruddha	- Contolled

Vikshepas	- There are several distractions (vikshepas) or obstacles on the path of Yoga.
Vyadhi	- Illness
Styana	- Idleness
Samshaya	- Doubt
Pramada	- Carelessness
Alasya	- Laziness
Dukha	- Unhappiness
Daurmansya	- Despair
Angamejayatva	- Unsteadiness of the body
Shvasa-Parashavas	- Unsteadiness of the breath

Means for Overcoming Obstacles

There are several means by which one can overcome problems and obstacles on the path of Yoga such as the practice of Ashtanga Yoga.

Besides one should cultivate the qualities mentioned below:

Maitri	- Friendliness
Karuna	- Kindness, compassion
Mudita	- Delight, joy
Upeksha	- Equanimity (in a hopeless situation), detachment

Abhyasa and Vairagya - Abhyasa means constant practice. Patanjali says that abhyasa must be done for a long duration, uninterrupted and with devotion. Also it must be done with faith, courage, memory, contemplation and awareness.

Vairagya is absence of wordly desires.

SALUTATIONS TO THE SUN.
(Surya Namaskar)

While performing the Sun Salutation Poses the different names of Lord Surya, the Sun God, may be recited (one name per cycle). The names, or mantras, which may be recited are as follows:

Mitraya namah
Ravaye namah
Suryaya namah
Bhanave namah
Khagaya namah
Pusne namah
Hiranyagarbhaya namah
Marichaye namah
Adityaya namah
Savitre namah
Akarya namah
Bhaskaraya namah

AUM

AUM is the mystic syllable and chant of the yogis. It is symbolic of creation, preservation, destruction or past, present, future. It is also called Pranava.

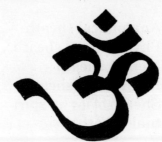

NDEX

sanas in Alphabetical Order